Concepts
of
Original Medicine

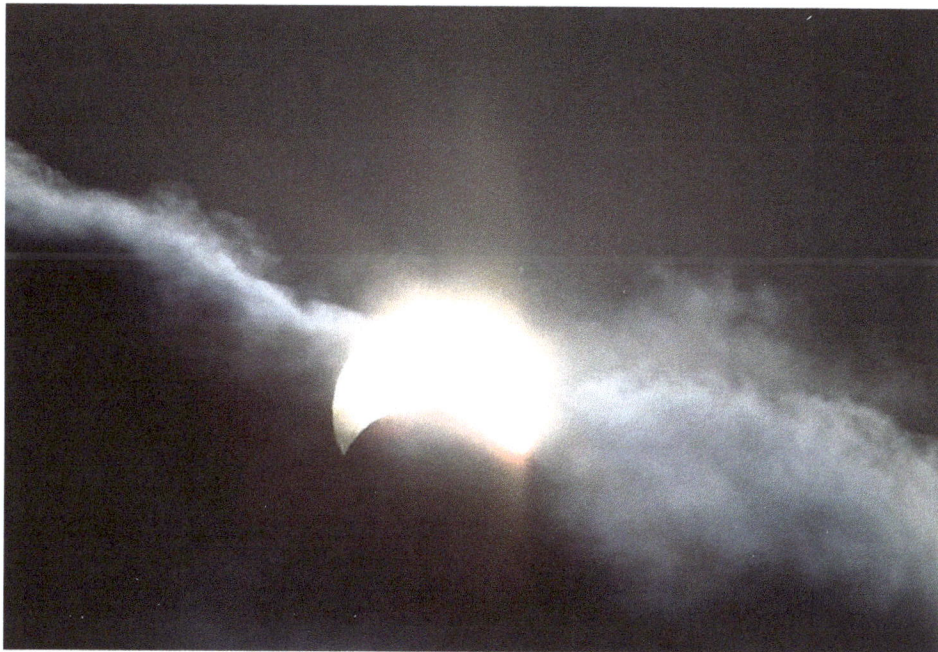

Jim Sharps, N.D., H.D., Dr. NSc., Ph.D.

Copyright © 2003, 2013, 2024 Jim Sharps, N.D., H.D., Dr. NSc., Ph.D.

Copyright © 2024 TEACH Services, Inc.

ISBN-13: 978-1-4796-1696-1 (Paperback)

ISBN-13: 978-1-4796-1788-3 (Spiral)

ISBN-13: 978-1-4796-1697-8 (ePub)

Library of Congress Control Number: 2024911200

All Scripture references marked (ASV) are taken from the American Standard Version of the Bible. Public domain.

All Scripture references marked (KJV) are taken from the King James Version of the Bible. Public domain.

All Scripture references marked (NKJV) are taken from the New King James Version® of the Bible, copyright © 1982 by Thomas Nelson. Used by permission. All rights reserved.

If you wish to contact the author for more information, visit https://iiomonline.org/

Printed by

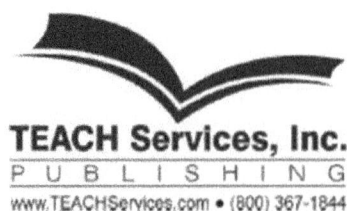

TEACH Services, Inc.
PUBLISHING
www.TEACHServices.com • (800) 367-1844

DEDICATION

This book, the college and faculty of the International Institute of Original Medicine (IIOM), and the educational concepts of the IIOM curriculum are dedicated to the glory and healing power of the Great Physician.

I wish to thank several people for their strong support, untiring efforts, and hard work that have resulted in transforming this Institute into a college that embraces the highest standards of academic excellence. Their efforts have enabled us to confidently seek accreditation of our programs for the benefit of our valued students.

To the following people, I owe a debt of gratitude that is beyond price:

Dr. Elisa Sharps

David Sharps

Dr. Linda Corbin

Susan Turley

Dr. Jim Duke

Drs. Duane and Nancy McEndree

Each one of the above-named individuals has given unselfishly and, in his or her own unique way, played a part in developing the content and quality of the IIOM program offerings.

And finally, to our valued students, I dedicate this book and wish you all the very best of health, happiness, and God's richest blessings as you pursue your personal health and professional objectives.

TABLE OF CONTENTS

PREFACE

"Blessed" with Poor Health - What a blessing it turned out to be when I was gifted poor health! This sounds like a strange statement to make, but I can't imagine pursuing the field of natural health if I had enjoyed superior health during my formative years.

For most of my childhood and adolescence, and during most of my twenty-four years working at IBM, I experienced poor health. This manifested itself in a variety of conditions, including allergies, gastrointestinal problems, lower back problems, chronic respiratory problems, skin problems, and general feelings of just not feeling right without having any specific names to describe these symptoms. Since I didn't know any better, I just assumed that this was normal.

My dad, who was an amateur health enthusiast and weightlifter, informally introduced me to the concepts of natural health. He extolled the powers of garlic, honey, whole wheat bread, and several other "health" foods. With my aversion to needles, hospitals, drugs and their possible side effects, as well as a case of what might be labeled "white coat syndrome", I initially ventured into alternative health protocols in my mid-twenties. I enjoyed watching TV programs about health, attended several free seminars on conventional and alternative health topics, and found myself drawn more and more into the depth and breadth of alternative health topics.

Eventually, the whole area of health and wellness became a passion and a hobby. Formally and informally, I began voraciously studying and practicing everything I could find on Eastern Medicine, Western Medicine, and "everything in between" regarding health, religion, and philosophy. While still at IBM, I learned and practiced massage, earned a certificate in acupressure, and earned several certificates or seriously participated in various diet and lifestyle programs. I also studied Buddhism, Hinduism, Islam, Taoism, and several other religions and philosophies.

By the time I was forty, I became more and more committed to natural health principles. In addition to experiencing improvements in my own health, I was enthusiastically sharing the concepts, principles, and practices I learned with family, friends, and anyone who would listen. I remember an incident when one of my friends asked me a simple question about blood pressure and, after a nonstop monologue on diet, lifestyle, herbs, and other aspects of the topic, I paused to take a breath and the person slipped in the still-resonating remark, "Wow, that was like asking what time it is and being told how to build a watch."

Now fast forward to my mid-to-late forties. I was experiencing conflict between pursuing my aspirations for executive management in the information technology field and my growing, insatiable passion for natural health. At that time, I was again blessed with corporate downsizing and its attendant stresses that occurred in the information technology field in general and at IBM in particular. The downsizing relieved me of my management responsibilities and, even though I was offered several opportunities to get back into executive management, I accepted an attractive severance package. After that, I pursued more structured and advanced educational opportunities in health and alternative medicine. I received my first doctoral degree from a California-based distance learning school in my late forties, and the rest is history.

During that time, I also developed a renewed connection with the Master Healer (I left formal religion for more than thirty years shortly after spending two years in the seminary, but that's another story to be left for another time) and was re-baptized in 1993.

I tell this story for two reasons: First, to make the point that a formal career in the natural health field was not even on my radar screen until my late forties when most people in my field were honing their education and experience to begin the most productive and lucrative years of their careers. So, for those of you, our valued students, who are coming to IIOM to begin a second career in midlife, I can personally attest that just such a life change is not only possible, but it is rewarding, enriching, and fulfilling! Secondly, and even more importantly, I told you my life story to emphasize that we can look at the events in our lives as *challenges* with the attendant negative stresses or as *opportunities* to walk in faith, learning the empowerment that comes from trust in and obedience to the laws of the all-powerful Creator and Sustainer of the heavens and the earth. I have learned and continue to learn that everything is a *mystery* until you turn it over to the Lord and that everything is a *victory* when you turn it over to the Lord.

I look forward with enthusiastic anticipation to the opportunity of working with our dynamic faculty at the International Institute of Original Medicine under the guidance of the Master Healer. Our goal is to provide content-rich, relevant, and empowering educational offerings for our valued students and health partners. My prayer is that your association with IIOM will prove to be a blessing to you and that you will come to know that His purpose for you is fulfilled with empowerment in your life and endeavors. On behalf of all of us at IIOM, I wish you health, happiness, and God's richest blessings as you pursue your personal health and professional goals.

JIM SHARPS, N.D., H.D., DR. NSC., PH.D.

INTRODUCTION

There are many ways of practicing the healing arts. At the International Institute of Original Medicine (IIOM), we recognize the tremendous task involved in setting down any instructions to do with health and the rules of right living. There have been thousands of volumes written, as well as many theories, valuable perspectives, advice, and counsel on these prodigious topics. All of them are well intentioned but provide varying levels of the truth. Our purpose is to present a powerful set of time-honored concepts, principles, and techniques for optimum health and wellness.

The original medicine concept can most closely be identified with the study of naturopathy, which focuses on the curative powers of nature. Naturopathy recognizes the sheer complexity of the human organism while at the same time appreciating the very powerful aspects of the simple laws that govern health and well-being. The original medicine concept differentiates itself from other schools of naturopathy that are not in harmony with original medicine principles. Many of these schools emphasize and promote concepts and principles with innate powers that are divorced and independent of a loving and creative force. The original medicine concept asserts that the Creator and Author of life originated and constantly enables the powerful and mysterious healing attributes found in nature.

Our intent at IIOM is to provide health education that is in harmony with the Creator's natural laws of health. We believe that our offerings provide our students, both Christian and non-Christian, with a powerful set of time-honored principles and techniques for developing the whole person - body, mind, and spirit.

Whatever principles of original medicine—in harmony with the Creator's plan for healthful living—are promoted by IIOM? It is the purpose of this book to answer that question. We do not intend to say that we have all the answers, but we want to share with you a foundational set of concepts, principles, and perspectives that support the original medicine viewpoint. It is our hope that this will enable and encourage you to carefully consider and evaluate this body of knowledge with an eye towards developing a personalized, well-thought-out philosophy and practice of health and healing.

To help our valued students develop this personalized and enriched perspective on health and healing, this book presents the following material:

1. The foundational basis for the original medicine approach to health and healing.
2. An appreciation for the conventional view of health in order to promote competence and relevance in addressing today's health concerns.
3. An emphasis on the importance of dealing with the whole person - body, mind, and spirit.

4. An emphasis on the classical aspects of the healing powers provided from the origins of man and an understanding of how true healing embraces an integrated and comprehensive application of time-honored laws of natural healing. This includes availing ourselves of the **eight natural wonders of the *natural health world*:**

   - fresh, pure air
   - pure, unadulterated water
   - the sun's healing energy
   - live, natural foods that are organic and that promote the life force within us
   - regular exercise for stimulation of the body's muscles, organs, and systems
   - rest for replenishing and regenerating our systemic resources
   - moderation and self-restraint
   - a belief and trust in Divine power, and the pursuance of a higher spiritual life.

We have been provided with these eight wonders by an all-wonderful and powerful Creator. After providing these wonders at the beginning of time, He has enabled the body to heal itself when it is in harmony with His moral and natural laws of health.

As competing, overlapping, and sometimes confusing and contradictory theories and perspectives on health emerge in the twenty-first century, we at IIOM are energized with the opportunity to equip and empower our valued students with the most powerful health system known to man—that of the original medicine perspective on total health of the body, mind, and spirit. Let us now go back to the origins of this life-enhancing system and lay the groundwork for your own personal and professional enrichment in original medicine.

CHAPTER ONE
THE "ORIGINAL" STORY

This chapter describes the foundation, beginnings, and origins of the original medicine concept. In her book *Patriarchs and Prophets*, Ellen G. White gives an inspirational and eloquent portrayal of the beginning: our earth's awesome beauty, power, and majesty; man's original, perfect created state; and the changed state of the earth and man that resulted from a breakdown in the moral and natural laws. The following excerpts, from her book based on Genesis chapters 1 and 2 in the Bible, lay a firm foundation for the original medicine concept.

THE CREATION STORY

"By the word of the Lord were the heavens made; and all the host of them by the breath of His mouth. For He spoke, and it was; He commanded, and it stood fast." (Psalm 33:6, 9) As the earth came forth from the hand of its Maker, it was exceedingly beautiful. Its surface was diversified with mountains, hills, and plains, interspersed with noble rivers and lovely lakes; but the hills and mountains were not abrupt and rugged, abounding in terrific steeps and frightful chasms, as they now do; the sharp, ragged edges of earth's rocky framework were buried beneath the fruitful soil, which everywhere produced a luxuriant growth of verdure. There were no loathsome swamps or barren deserts. Graceful shrubs and delicate flowers greeted the eye at every turn. The heights were crowned with trees more majestic than any that now exist. The air, untainted by foul miasma, was clear and healthful. The entire landscape outshone in beauty the decorated grounds of the proudest palace. The angelic host viewed the scene with delight and rejoiced at the wonderful works of God.

After the earth with its teeming animal and vegetable life had been called into existence, man, the crowning work of the Creator, and the one for whom the beautiful earth had been fitted up, was brought upon the stage of action. He was given dominion over all that his eye could behold; for "God said, Let Us make man in Our image, after Our likeness: and let them have dominion over . . . all the earth … So, God created man in His own image; . . . male and female created He them."

---

[1]White, Ellen G. *Patriarchs and Prophets*. (Review and Herald Publishing Association, 1958).

Here is clearly set forth the origin of the human race; and the divine record is so plainly stated that there is no occasion for erroneous conclusions. God created man in His own image. Here is no mystery. There is no ground for the supposition that man was evolved by slow degrees of development from the lower forms of animal or vegetable life. Such teaching lowers the great work of the Creator to the level of man's narrow, earthly conceptions. Men are so intent upon excluding God from the sovereignty of the universe that they degrade man and defraud him of the dignity of his origin. He who set the starry worlds on high and tinted with delicate skill the flowers of the field, who filled the earth and the heavens with the wonders of His power, when He came to crown His glorious work, to place one in the midst to stand as ruler of the fair earth, did not fail to create a being worthy of the hand that gave him life. The genealogy of our race, as given by inspiration, traces back its origin, not to a line of developing germs, mollusks, and quadrupeds, but to the great Creator. Though formed from the dust, Adam was "the son of God."

Man was to bear God's image, both in outward resemblance and in character. Christ alone is "the express image" (Hebrews 1:3) of the Father; but man was formed in the likeness of God. His nature was in harmony with the will of God. His mind was capable of comprehending divine things. His affections were pure; his appetites and passions were under the control of reason. He was holy and happy in bearing the image of God and in perfect obedience to His will.

As man came forth from the hand of his Creator, he was of lofty stature and perfect symmetry. His countenance bore the ruddy tint of health and glowed with the light of life and joy. Adam's height was much greater than that of men who now inhabit the earth. Eve was somewhat less in stature; yet her form was noble, and full of beauty. The sinless pair wore no artificial garments; they were clothed with a covering of light and glory, such as the angels wear. So long as they lived in obedience to God, this robe of light continued to enshroud them.

Everything that God had made was the perfection of beauty, and nothing seemed wanting that could contribute to the happiness of the holy pair; yet the Creator gave them still another token of His love, by preparing a garden especially for their home. In this garden were trees of every variety, many of them laden with fragrant and delicious fruit. There were lovely vines, growing upright, yet presenting a most graceful appearance, with their branches drooping under their load of tempting fruit of the richest and most varied hues. It was the work of Adam and Eve to train the branches of the vine to form bowers, thus making for themselves a dwelling from living trees covered with foliage and fruit. There were fragrant flowers of every hue in rich profusion. In the midst of the garden stood the tree of life, surpassing in glory all other trees. Its fruit appeared like apples of gold and silver and had the power to perpetuate life.

The creation was now complete. "The heavens and the earth were finished, and all the host of them." "And God saw everything that He had made, and behold, it was very good." (Genesis 2:1, 1:31) Eden bloomed on earth. Adam and Eve had free access to the tree of life. No taint of sin or shadow of death marred the fair creation.

The great Jehovah had laid the foundations of the earth; He had dressed the whole world in the garb of beauty and had filled it with things useful to man; He had created all the wonders of the land and of the sea. In six days the great work of creation had been accomplished. And God "rested on the seventh day from all His work which He had made. And God blessed the seventh day and sanctified it: because that in it He had rested from all His work which God created and made." (Genesis 2:2, 3) God looked with satisfaction upon the work of His hands. All was perfect, worthy of its divine Author, and He rested, not as one weary, but as well pleased with the fruits of His wisdom and goodness and the manifestations of His glory.

After resting upon the seventh day, God sanctified it, or set it apart, as a day of rest for man. Following the example of the Creator, man was to rest upon this sacred day, that as he should look upon the heavens and the earth, he might reflect upon God's great work of creation; and that as he should behold the evidences of God's wisdom and goodness, his heart might be filled with love and reverence for his Maker. Nature speaks to man's senses, declaring that there is a living God, the Creator, the Supreme Ruler of all. The beauty that clothes the earth is a token of God's love. We may behold it in the everlasting hills, in the lofty trees, in the opening buds and the delicate flowers. All speak to us of God. The Sabbath, ever pointing to Him who made them all, bids men open the great book of nature and trace therein the wisdom, the power, and the love of the Creator.

God gave man noble traits of character, with no bias toward evil. He endowed him with high intellectual powers and presented before him the strongest possible inducements to be true to his allegiance. Obedience, perfect and perpetual, was the condition of eternal happiness. On this condition he was to have access to the tree of life.

The home of our first parents was to be a pattern for other homes as their children should go forth to occupy the earth. That home, beautified by the hand of God Himself, was not a gorgeous palace. Men, in their pride, delight in magnificent and costly edifices and glory in the works of their own hands; but God placed Adam in a garden. This was his dwelling. The blue heavens were its dome; the earth, with its delicate flowers and carpet of living green, was its floor; and the leafy branches of the goodly trees were the canopy. Its walls were hung with the most magnificent adornment--the handiwork of the great Master Artist. In the surroundings of the holy pair was a lesson for all time—the lesson that true happiness is found, not in the indulgence of pride and luxury, but in communion with God through His created works. If men would give less attention to the artificial, and would cultivate greater simplicity, they would come far nearer to answering the purpose of God in their creation. Pride and ambition are never satisfied, but those who are truly wise will find substantial and elevating pleasure in the sources of enjoyment that God has placed within the reach of all.

To the dwellers in Eden was committed the care of the garden, 'to dress it and to keep it.' Their occupation was not wearisome, but pleasant and invigorating. God appointed labor as a blessing to man, to occupy his mind, to strengthen his body, and to develop his faculties. In mental and physical activity, Adam found one of the highest pleasures of his holy existence.

The holy pair were not only children under the fatherly care of God but students receiving instruction from the all-wise Creator. They were visited by angels, and were granted communion with their Maker, with no obscuring veil between. They were full of the vigor imparted by the tree of life, and their intellectual power was but little less than that of the angels. The mysteries of the visible universe — 'the wondrous works of Him which is perfect in knowledge' (Job 37:16) -- afforded them an exhaustless source of instruction and delight. The laws and operations of nature that have engaged men's study for six thousand years were opened to their minds by the infinite Framer and Upholder of all. They held conversations with leaf and flower and tree, gathering from each the secrets of its life. The order and harmony of creation spoke to them of infinite wisdom and power. They were ever discovering some attraction that filled their hearts with deeper love and called forth fresh expressions of gratitude.

So long as they remained loyal to the divine law, their capacity to know, to enjoy, and to love would continually increase. They would be constantly gaining new treasures of knowledge, discovering fresh springs of happiness, and obtaining clearer and yet clearer conceptions of the immeasurable, unfailing love of God.

Our first parents, though created innocent and holy, were not placed beyond the possibility of wrongdoing. God made them free moral agents, capable of appreciating the wisdom and benevolence of His character and the justice of His requirements, and with full liberty to yield or to withhold obedience. They were to enjoy communion with God and with holy angels; but before they could be rendered eternally secure, their loyalty must be tested. At the very beginning of man's existence, a check was placed upon the desire for self-indulgence. The tree of knowledge, which stood near the tree of life in the midst of the garden, was to be a test of the obedience, faith, and love of our parents. While permitted to eat freely of every other tree, they were forbidden to taste the fruit of the tree of knowledge on pain of death.

And when, as a result of disobedience, man was driven from his beautiful home, and forced to struggle with a stubborn soil to gain his daily bread, that very labor, although widely different from his pleasant occupation in the garden, was a safeguard against temptation and a source of happiness.

SUMMARY AND CONCLUSIONS

Thus, man and all created things in the world were perfect in every way. There was a powerful simplicity and integrity that governed our beginnings. The natural treasures that were established at the dawn of humanity have withstood the test of time, even to this current day, as the most powerful system of health, longevity, and happiness. For the prevention and reversal of disease, our best opportunity is to be in harmony with these immutable laws.

Many of the health systems today provide varying degrees of the elements of the original prescription for health and vitality. To the extent that they are in harmony with the original principles, they enjoy their greatest opportunity for effectiveness. Our health status is also amenable to these same principles, and concepts. These principles are not man-made, nor has man demonstrated any ability to improve on them.

Original medicine takes us back to our roots and encourages us to rediscover the power and simplicity of the "Original Medicine" eight wonders of the world for maximizing our potential. We are made by a loving Creator who provided us with everything we need from the beginning of time to enjoy a profoundly happy existence on this planet. Knowledge and application of His laws gives us a standard for evaluating other health systems and modalities.

I believe that the description of the "original" story lays a foundation for understanding a powerful set of principles for maximizing our potential. Our objective at the International Institute of Original Medicine is to provide relevant course material for tapping into the most powerful Source of wisdom in the universe.

THE CONDITION OF THE EARTH BEFORE AND AFTER THE FLOOD

The following excerpts from *Patriarchs and Prophets* (and based on Genesis chapters 6 and 7 in the Bible) describe the degeneration of man from his original perfect state.

In the days of Noah, a double curse was resting upon the earth in consequence of Adam's transgression and of the murder committed by Cain. Yet this had not greatly changed the face of nature. There were evident tokens of decay, but the earth was still rich and beautiful in the gifts of God's providence. The hills were crowned with majestic trees supporting the fruit-laden branches of the vine. The vast, gardenlike plains were clothed with verdure, and sweet with the fragrance of a thousand flowers. The fruits of the earth were in great variety, and almost without limit. The trees far surpassed in size, beauty, and perfect proportion any now to be found; their wood was of fine grain and hard substance, closely resembling stone, and hardly less enduring. Gold, silver, and precious stones existed in abundance.

13

The human race yet retained much of its early vigor. Only a few generations had passed since Adam had had access to the tree of life in the Garden of Eden, which had prolonged life, and so man's existence was still measured by centuries. Had that long-lived people, with their rare powers to plan and execute, devoted themselves to the service of God, they would have made their Creator's name a praise in the earth and would have answered the purpose for which He gave them life. But they failed to do this. There were many giants, men of great stature and strength, renowned for wisdom, skillful in devising the most cunning and wonderful works; but their guilt in giving in to iniquity was in proportion to their skill and mental ability.

God bestowed upon those who lived before the Flood many and rich gifts; but they used His bounties to glorify themselves and turned them into a curse by fixing their affections upon the gifts instead of the Giver.

Men put God out of their knowledge and worshiped the creatures of their own imagination; and as the result, they became more and more debased. It is a law of the human mind that by beholding we become changed. Man will rise no higher than his conceptions of truth, purity, and holiness. If the mind is never exalted above the level of humanity, if it is not uplifted by faith to contemplate infinite wisdom and love, then man will be constantly sinking lower and lower. 'God saw that the wickedness of man was great in the earth, and that every imagination of the thoughts of his heart was only evil continuously. The earth also was corrupt before God; and the earth was filled with violence.' God had given men His commandments as a rule of life, but His law was transgressed, and every conceivable sin was the result. The wickedness of men was open and daring, justice was trampled in the dust, and the cries of the oppressed reached unto heaven.

Crime and wretchedness rapidly increased. Men exulted in their deeds of violence. They delighted in destroying the life of animals; and the use of flesh for food rendered them still more cruel and bloodthirsty, until they came to regard human life with astonishing indifference.

The world was in its infancy; yet iniquity had become so deep and widespread that God could no longer bear with it; and He said, 'I will destroy man whom I have created from the face of the earth.' He declared that His Spirit should not always strive with the guilty race. If they did not cease to pollute the world and its rich treasures, then He would blot them from His creation and would destroy the things with which He had delighted to bless them. He would sweep away the beasts of the field and the vegetation that furnished such an abundant supply of food. He would transform the fair earth into one vast scene of desolation and ruin.

A hundred and twenty years before the Flood, the Lord, by a holy angel declared to Noah His purpose, and directed him to build an ark. While building the ark he was to preach that God would bring a flood of water upon the earth to destroy the wicked. Those who would believe the message and would prepare for that event by repentance and reformation, should find pardon and be saved. God gave Noah the exact dimensions of the ark and explicit directions regarding its construction in every particular. Human wisdom could not have devised a structure of so great strength and durability. God was the designer, and Noah the master builder.

"By faith Noah, being warned of God of things not seen as yet, moved with fear, prepared an ark to the saving of his house; by the which he condemned the world, and became heir of the righteousness which is by faith." (Hebrews 11:7) While Noah was giving his warning message to the world, his works testified of his sincerity. It was thus that his faith was perfected and made evident. He gave the world an example of believing just what God says.

For centuries the laws of nature had been fixed. The recurring seasons had come in their order. Before this, rain had never fallen; the earth had been watered by a mist or dew. The rivers had never yet passed their boundaries. Those who lived before the Flood reasoned that nature was above the God of nature, and that nature's laws were so firmly established that God Himself could not change them. They asserted that if there were any truth in what Noah had said, the men of renown--the wise, the prudent, the great men--would have understood this matter.

But it was not multitudes or majorities that were on the side of right. Noah was regarded as a wild fanatic, but he stood like a rock amid the tempest. Surrounded by popular contempt and ridicule, he distinguished himself by his holy integrity and unwavering faithfulness.

Noah had faithfully followed the instructions that he had received from God. The ark was finished in every part as the Lord had directed, and was stored with food for man and beast. And now the servant of God made his last solemn appeal to the people. Again, they rejected his words. Suddenly a silence fell upon the mocking throng. Beasts of every description, the fiercest as well as the most gentle, were seen coming from mountain and forest and quietly making their way toward the ark. A noise as of a rushing wind was heard, and lo, birds were flocking from all directions, their numbers darkening the heavens, and in perfect order they passed to the ark. Animals obeyed the command of God, while men were disobedient.

For seven days after Noah and his family entered the ark, there appeared no sign of the coming storm. But upon the eighth day dark clouds overspread the heavens. Soon large drops of rain began to fall. The world had never witnessed anything like this, and the hearts of men were struck with fear. Then the fountains of the great deep were broken up, and the windows of heaven were opened. Water came from the clouds in mighty torrents. Rivers broke away from their boundaries and overflowed the valleys. Jets of water burst from the earth with indescribable force, throwing massive rocks hundreds of feet into the air. As the violence of the storm increased, trees, buildings, rocks, and earth were hurled in every direction. The terror of man and beast was beyond description.

"By the word of God . . . the world that then was, being overflowed with water, perished. . ." (2 Peter 3:5-7) Love, no less than justice, demanded that God's judgments should put a check on sin. Said Christ, "As in the days that were before the Flood they were eating and drinking, marrying and giving in marriage, until the day that Noah entered into the ark, and knew not until the Flood came, and took them all away. . ." (Matthew 24:38, 39) God did not condemn those who lived before the Flood for eating and drinking; He had given them the fruits of the earth in great abundance to supply their physical wants. Their sin consisted in taking these gifts without gratitude to the Giver, and debasing themselves by indulging appetite without restraint.

A similar condition of things exists now. That which is lawful is carried to excess. Appetite is indulged without restraint. Intemperance numbs the moral and spiritual powers and prepares the way for indulgence of the lower passions. The spirit of anarchy is permeating all nations, and the outbreaks that from time to time excite the horror of the world are but indications of the pent-up fires of passion and lawlessness that, having once escaped control, will fill the earth with woe and desolation. The view of the world before the Flood represents the apparent condition of modern society.

SUMMARY AND CONCLUSIONS

Knowledge of the Creation and the subsequent flood should give us an appreciation for the massive changes that took place in the earth's natural resources and the accompanying changes in our health potential. Even though the earth's resources were compromised, the original laws of health remain the most powerful health system available for maximizing our potential. There were many scoffers in Noah's time, and we still have many scoffers today. The scientific viewpoint in the days of Noah was that it never rained and as a result many refused the invitation to climb on board the ark.

Today a similar condition exists, in that there are so many vehicles presented for getting us to reach our health goals. This results in both confusion and ineffective modalities and systems. In our post-flood existence climbing on the boat is still the safest and most effective way of achieving outrageous health and vitality. Simply stated, climbing on the original medicine boat is the best way to keep our feet on dry ground and protect ourselves from being deluged with a myriad of watered-down and ship-wrecked health systems and modalities.

CHAPTER TWO
THE "ORIGINAL" DIET

This chapter describes what the Creator provided as man's original diet to consist of and how and why the eating of animals began. The following excerpts are adapted from the book *Counsels on Diet and Foods* by Ellen G. White[1].

In order to know what the best foods are, we must study God's original plan for man's diet that was given to us at creation in the Garden of Eden. Our Creator understands our dietary needs and appointed Adam his food. "Then God said, Behold, I have given you every plant yielding seed, . . . and every tree which has fruit yielding seed; it shall be food for you." (Genesis 1:29) Even the animals themselves were not created to eat other animals. "To every beast of the earth and to every bird of the sky, and to everything that moves on the earth which has life I have given every green plant for food." (Genesis 1:30) After man had to leave the Garden of Eden, the ground brought forth "thorns and thistles." Man had to gain his livelihood by tilling the earth, and he received permission to eat also "the herb of the field." (Genesis 3:18)

Fruits, vegetables, nuts, seeds, and grains constitute the diet chosen for us by our Creator. These foods, prepared in as simple and natural a manner as possible, are the most healthful and nourishing. They impart strength, power of endurance, and vigor of intellect that are not afforded by a more complex and stimulating diet. The diet appointed man in the beginning did not include animal food. Not until after the flood, when every green thing on the earth had been destroyed, did man receive permission to eat flesh.

It was contrary to the original plan to have the life of any creature taken. There was to be no death in Eden. The fruit of the trees in the Garden of Eden was the food best suited to meet man's dietary requirements. God gave man no permission to eat animal food until after the Flood. Everything had been destroyed upon which man could subsist, and therefore, the Lord gave Noah permission to eat of the clean animals that he had taken with him into the ark. But animal food was not the healthiest article of food for man.

When God led the children of Israel out of Egypt, it was His purpose to establish them in the land of Canaan a pure, happy, healthy people. He subjected them to a course of discipline, which, had it been cheerfully followed, would have resulted in good, both to themselves and to their posterity. He removed flesh-food from them in a great measure. He had granted them flesh in answer to their clamors, just before reaching Sinai, but it was furnished for only one day. God might have provided flesh as easily as manna, but a restriction was placed upon the people for their good. It was His purpose to supply them with food better suited to their wants than the feverish diet to which many of them had

1   White, Ellen G. *Counsels on Diet and Foods* (Review and Herald Publishing Association, 1938).

been accustomed in Egypt. The perverted appetite was to be brought into a healthier state, that they might enjoy the food originally provided for man--the fruits of the earth, which God gave to Adam and Eve in Eden.

Nowhere can we find a better illustration of dietary temperance and the blessings it brings than in the Bible story of Daniel and his companions. These Hebrew youth were taken captive to the city of Babylon. Even there, none could match them. Their erect form, firm, elastic step, fair countenance, undimmed senses, and untainted breath—all certificates of good health—showed their obedience to God's laws of health. In their training in Babylon, they were admitted to the king's palace and told they should eat the meat and drink the wine that came from the king's table. In all this, the king considered that he was not only showing great honor to them, but also securing for his service their best physical and mental development. Here Daniel was brought to a severe test. Should he adhere to the teachings of his fathers and of God concerning food? This would offend the king and he would probably lose not only his position but also his life. Or should be disregard the commandments of the Lord and retain the favor of the king. Daniel decided to stand firmly for the Lord. "He purposed in his heart that he would not defile himself with the portion of the king's meat nor with the wine which the king drank." (Daniel 1:8) Daniel made a request that he and his companions not be required to eat the king's food for ten days, but only be given "some vegetables and water," and he was given permission to do this. "At the end of ten days, their appearances seemed better, and they were fatter than all the youths who had eaten the king's choice food." (Daniel 1:12, 15)

Our danger is not from scarcity of food, but from abundance. We are constantly tempted to excess. All our habits, tastes, and inclinations must be educated to be in harmony with God's laws of life and health. God always honors the right, but God will not intervene to preserve men from the consequences of violating His health laws.

SUMMARY AND CONCLUSIONS

Fruits, vegetables, nuts, seeds, and grains constitute the diet chosen for us by our Creator. After man left the Garden of Eden, herbs were added to the diet as the soil grew weeds and everything became more difficult to cultivate. If the use of flesh foods had been essential to health and strength, animal food would have been included in the original diet given to man in the beginning. When the flood took away all vegetation, God did allow men to eat meat. When God led the children of Israel out of Egypt, they were used to eating meat. In that journey, they complained, and God briefly gave them quail to eat. However, their everyday food was manna supplied by God. Daniel and his friends, captives of Babylon, showed that the original diet is still the best when they ate vegetables and water for ten days and still physically surpassed other youth who ate the meat, wine, and sweets of the king.

One of the biggest challenges practitioners of original medicine face today in dealing with chronic degenerative diseases is how to help people overcome the effects of poor dietary choices. IIOM original medicine courses are designed to present information on proper dietary choices as well as practical strategies for overcoming the effects of compromised dietary practices. IIOM courses refute many of the popular myths and misconceptions about dietary practices and present evidence-based solutions that show the awesome power of a vegetarian diet. A vegetarian diet is not only a powerful approach to preventing and reversing disease processes, it also enhances athletic, mental, and spiritual attributes and capacities. The original diet still provides the highest level oof vitality, health, and wellness to this very day.

CHAPTER THREE
THE "ORIGINAL" SCHOOLS

This chapter describes the education of man in the Garden of Eden and later after sin entered the world. The role of a Supreme Being who is the Creator and Educator of man is a theme that reinforces the foundational concepts of original medicine. The following excerpts are from *Counsels on Education*[1] (based on Genesis 1 and 2) and *Patriarchs and Prophets* (and based on 1 Samuel 3 through 7).

In the Garden of Eden, God personally directed the education of Adam and Eve.

Eden was the schoolroom, nature was the lesson book, the Creator Himself was the Instructor, and the parents of the human race were the students. God's glory in the heavens, the innumerable worlds in their orderly revolutions, the mysteries of light and sound, of day and night—all of these were open to the study of our first parents. On every leaf of the forest or stone of the mountains, in every shining star, in earth and air and sky, God's name was written. The order and harmony of creation taught them of His infinite wisdom and power. Adam was acquainted with the nature and habits of every living creature, and he named them all.

Ten generations of man after the Flood, God chose Abraham to become the father of the Hebrews, a people who were to be the teachers and examples to all of God's children everywhere. The Lord Himself directed their education. His care was not restricted to their religion alone; whatever affected their mental or physical well-being was also the subject of divine providence.

God had commanded the Hebrews to teach their children His laws and requirements and to make them acquainted with all His dealings with their fathers. This was one of the special duties of every parent--one that was not to be delegated to another. Thoughts of God were to be associated with all the events of daily life. The great truths of God's providence and of the future life were to be impressed on the young mind. It was to be trained to see God in the scenes of nature and the words of revelation. The stars of heaven, trees and flowers of the field, lofty mountains, flowing brooks--all spoke of the Creator.

The schools of the prophets were founded by Samuel the prophet to furnish the nation with men qualified to act in the reverence of God as leaders and counselors. The instructors were men not only well versed in divine truth, but those who had themselves enjoyed communion with God and had received the special endowment of His Spirit. They enjoyed the respect and confidence of the people, both for learning and

---

1   White, Ellen G. *Counsels on Education*. (Pacific Press Publishing Association, 1952).

piety. Samuel gathered young men who were pious, intelligent, and studious. As they communed with God and studied His word and His works, wisdom from above was added to their natural endowments. The pupils of these schools sustained themselves by their own labor in tilling the soil or in some useful labor.

The chief subjects of study in these schools were the law of God, the instructions given to Moses, sacred history, sacred music, and poetry. It was the object of all study to learn the will of God and man's duty toward Him. Not only were students taught the duty of prayer, they were also taught how to pray, how to approach their Creator, how to exercise faith in Him, and how to understand and obey the teachings of His Spirit.

All the various capabilities that men possess—the talents of mind and soul and body--are given to them by God. These capabilities are to be employed so as to reach the highest possible degree of excellence. But this cannot be done in a selfish and exclusive way; for the character of God, whose likeness we are to receive, is benevolence and love. Every faculty, every attribute with which the Creator has endowed us is to be employed for His glory and for the uplifting of our fellow men. Instead of appealing to pride and selfish ambition, kindling a spirit of emulation, teachers should endeavor to awaken the love for goodness and truth and beauty--to arouse the desire for excellence. Students should seek the development of God's gifts within themselves, not to excel others, but to fulfill the purpose of the Creator and to receive His likeness. Instead of being directed to mere earthly standards, or being actuated by the desire for self-exaltation, the mind should be directed to the Creator, to know Him and to become like Him.

"The fear of the Lord is the beginning of wisdom: and the knowledge of the Holy is understanding." (Proverbs 9:10) The great work of life is character building, and knowledge of God is the foundation of all true education. The law of God is a reflection of His character. Hence the psalmist says, "All Thy commandments are righteousness;" and "through Thy precepts I get understanding." (Psalm 119:172, 104) God has revealed Himself to us in His word and in the works of creation. Through the volume of inspiration and the book of nature we are to obtain knowledge of God.

It is a law of the mind that it gradually adapts itself to the subjects upon which it dwells. As an educating power, the Bible is without equal. In the word of God, the mind finds subject for the deepest thought, the loftiest aspiration. The Bible is the most instructive history that men possess. It came from the fountain of eternal truth, and a divine hand has preserved its purity through all the ages. It lights up the far-distant past, where human research seeks vainly to penetrate. In God's word we behold the power that laid the foundation of the earth and that stretched out the heavens. Only in the Bible can we find a history of man that is not contaminated by human prejudice or human pride. The curtain that separates the visible from the invisible world is lifted, and we behold the conflict of the opposing forces of good and evil, from the first entrance of sin to the final triumph of righteousness and truth. In the contemplation of the truths presented in His word, the mind of the student is brought into communion with the Infinite Mind. Such a study not only refines and ennobles the character, but it expands and invigorates the mental powers.

The teachings of the Bible affect man's prosperity in all the relations of this life. The Bible unfolds principles that are the cornerstone of a nation's prosperity--principles that safeguard the family--principles without which no man can attain usefulness, happiness, and honor in this life and the hope of a future, immortal life. There is no position in life, no phase of human experience, for which the teaching of the Bible is not an essential preparation. Studied and obeyed, the word of God gives to the world men of stronger and more active intellect than will the most intense study of human philosophy. A study of the Bible produces men of strength and solid character with keen perception and sound judgment--men who honor God and are a blessing to the world.

In the study of the sciences, we are also to obtain knowledge of the Creator. All true science is but an interpretation of the handwriting of God in the natural world. Science brings from her research fresh evidence of the wisdom and power of God. Rightly understood, both science--as seen in the book of nature--and the Bible acquaint us with God and teach us of the wise and beneficent laws through which He works.

Students should be led to see God in all the works of creation. The Great Teacher drew illustrations from the familiar scenes of nature to simplify and deeply impress His teachings upon the minds of those who heard. The birds singing in the leafy branches, the flowers of the valley, the lofty trees, the fruitful lands, the springing grain, the barren soil, the setting sun filling the heavens with its beams--all served as means of instruction. He connected the visible works of the Creator with the words of life that He spoke, so that whenever these things were seen, those who heard him would remember the lessons of truth He had taught.

The lofty mountains, the fruitful valleys, the broad, deep ocean--these things of nature speak to man of his Creator's love. He has linked us to Himself by unnumbered tokens in heaven and in earth. "God is love," is written upon every opening bud, upon the petals of every flower, and upon every spire of grass. All things in nature testify to the tender, fatherly care of our God and to His desire to make His children happy. In all that He does He has the well-being of His children in view. He does not require them to give up anything that would be in their best interests to retain.

The Scripture says: "The fear of the Lord tends to life: and he that hath it shall abide satisfied." (Proverbs 19:23) "What man is he that desires life and many days, that he may see good? Depart from evil, and do good; seek peace, and pursue it." (Psalm 34:12-14) These words of wisdom "are life unto those that find them and health to all their flesh." (Proverbs 4:22)

True religion brings man into harmony with the laws of God—His physical, mental, and moral laws. True religion teaches self-control, serenity, and temperance. It ennobles the mind, refines the taste, and sanctifies the judgment. It makes the soul partake of the purity of heaven. Faith in God's love and overruling providence lightens the burdens of anxiety and care. It fills the heart with joy and contentment in the highest or the lowliest lot. Religion promotes health, lengthens life, and heightens our enjoyment of all its blessings. It opens to the soul a never-failing fountain of happiness. Man is doing the greatest injury and injustice to his own soul when he thinks and acts contrary to the will of God. No real joy can be found in that path. The path of transgression leads to misery and destruction; but wisdom's "ways are ways of pleasantness, and all her paths are peace." (Proverbs 3:17)

The physical as well as the religious training practiced in the schools of the Hebrews should be studied. It taught that there is an intimate relation between the mind and the body. In order to reach a high standard of moral and intellectual attainment, the laws that control our physical being must be heeded. To secure a strong, well-balanced character, both the mental and the physical powers must be exercised and developed. What study is more important than the study of these wonderful organisms--our bodies--that God has given to us and the study of the laws by which our bodies may be preserved in health?

Today as in years past, real success in education depends upon how faithfully men carry out the Creator's plan. The true object of education is to restore the image of God in the soul.

Day by day the wonderful works of God, the evidences of His wisdom and power in creating and sustaining the universe, the infinite mystery of love and wisdom in the plan of redemption, will open to the mind in new beauty. "Eye hath not seen, nor ear heard, neither have entered into the heart of man, the things which God hath prepared for them that love Him." (1 Corinthians 2:9) Even in this life we may catch glimpses of His presence and may taste the joy of communion with Heaven, but the fullness of its joy and blessing will be reached in the hereafter. Eternity alone can reveal the glorious destiny to which man, restored to God's image, may attain.

SUMMARY AND CONCLUSIONS

There is no greater source of knowledge and wisdom than the Original Provider of all created things. The foundational concepts and principles of the original schools offered students a powerful template for learning and mental advancement. When our learning is in harmony with the principles of true learning, we become more empowered to understand complex topics. Rather than trying to force-fit our observations into our ever-changing theories as we learn more and more about the subjects we study, we can see things more clearly and coherently.

Some important conclusions to be drawn from an appreciation of the original schools include the following:

- The laws of true science and religion are not in conflict with each other, and when they are in harmony with each other, understanding and wisdom reach their highest potential.
- Knowledge is not the property of any one man or institution to be used for selfish purposes.
- Knowledge is not uni-dimensional but incorporates the total integration of physical, mental, and spiritual aspects in the learning experience.
- All of our knowledge and talents are gifts that, when properly used, enable personal enrichment and multiply the enrichment of all mankind.
- Seeking first knowledge of the Original knowledge-giver is the most enabling and empowering road for expanding our mental and discerning capacities.

CHAPTER FOUR
MADE IN HIS OWN IMAGE

This chapter describes how the great Creator of the universe personally formed man from the ground and made a deliberate decision to make man as a reflection of the image of God. The complexity and marvelous design of the human body is also discussed.

"Then God said, Let us make man in Our image, after Our likeness…" (Genesis 1:26). And so the Lord formed the man from the ground and breathed into his nostrils the breath of life and man became a living soul." (Genesis 2:7). Man was made "in the image of God." There are many things in these Bible verses that help us to understand who we human beings really are. Let's review them:

First, we understand that God Himself made us in a separate and special act of creation. God's people, His masterpiece of creation, did not evolve from some lower kind of animal.

Second, we understand that God made us to be *different* from every other living thing. Our bodies were made from the elements found in the Earth, but we are still unique from any other form of life. The Bible tells us that God simply spoke "Let there be..," and the plants and animals came into existence, but God *personally* fashioned man's physical nature and body from the elements in the ground.

Third, the Bible plainly states that God chose to make human beings "in His own image and likeness." We were created as spiritual and physical beings after Our Heavenly Father's *likeness*. This is an important difference between human beings and animals. God created His children as special beings. God, in essence, created us to be *like Himself.*

You are the child of royalty! You are the magnificent work of the all-powerful Creator of the universe, the true originator of the species. There is none like you in this whole universe. God made you and fashioned you after His image. In God's message to mankind inscribed in the Bible, we are told that we were constructed with precision. "I will praise thee; for I am fearfully and wonderfully made: marvelous are thy works; and that my soul knows right well." (Psalm 139:14). Even though most the Bible passages clearly refer to the dignity of mankind, how many of us really appreciate how truly complex and perfect the body construction is?

OUR MARVELOUS BODIES

The human body is a true marvel, from the largest organ down to the workings of the tiniest molecules. Let's briefly consider some of the more familiar parts of the body and the miraculous work they perform on a daily basis.

On a microscopic level in the body, we encounter cells. Many people think of a cell as a relatively simple structure because it is so small. However, even a single cell is extremely and amazingly complex. According to Walter J. Veith, world-renowned anthropologist and nutritionist[1], the structure and function of the cell conclusively point to a deliberate design by a Creator and not to chance and random processes that occurred over vast periods of time. He notes that some scientists/evolutionists say that life could have begun on a planet with certain types of gases that, when hit with an electrical charge, form organic molecules. This can be demonstrated in the controlled environment of the laboratory, but these organic molecules immediately disintegrate, demonstrating that complex organisms could never come from this. In addition, the conditions needed to form amino acids are very different from the conditions needed to form simple sugars. So, the probability of the complexity of life arising in this manner is very remote. In addition, even if you somehow had many molecules of amino acids and simple sugars, they need to be arranged in long chains to begin to approximate life functions. Enzymes are required to form these long chains, but where would these enzymes come from? This question has never been satisfactorily answered by these scientists/evolutionists. In fact, laboratory experiments have never produced any chain molecule, let alone one as complex as DNA or RNA. Creationist scientists have estimated that the probability of forming a chain molecule such as DNA is about 1 to 10^{80}. At first glance, that number seems large, but not impossibly large. However, consider this. If you were to count all of the subatomic particles in the universe — not just all the stars, not just all the molecules, not just all the atoms — but all the subatomic particles that make up the atoms (neutrons, protons, electrons, quarks) — they would number less than 10^{80}. And so, for a single complex organic molecule to arise on its own means that it is more likely to occur than all the subatomic particles in the universe. In fact, Professor Veith illustrates the odds of forming a chain molecule of DNA are greater than the odds of somehow having New York City — with all of its billions of working machines and buildings and living people — suddenly appear out of nowhere. As Professor Veith notes, when faced with this dilemma, you have two choices. You can either believe that life originated by chance or by the intelligent design of a loving Creator.

On a macroscopic level in the body, we see the body organs and systems, all of which are unique and divinely fashioned.

---

1   Veith, Walter J. *The Genes of Genesis* DVD. Copyright Amazing Discoveries, 2004.

The adult heart is about the size of a fist and only weighs 0.5 to 0.75 pounds, and yet each day it pumps blood through about 60,000 miles of blood vessels. In fact, it pumps enough blood to fill a 2,000-gallon tanker car every day. In a lifetime, the heart can pump about 450,000 tons of blood. The heart does all this without our conscious control! In the average person, the heart contracts 72 times a minute, over 100,000 times a day, and over 37 million times a year. If the leg or arm muscles had to work as constantly as the heart muscle does, they would be exhausted in minutes. The heart pumps whether a person is awake or asleep. With exercise, it contracts more frequently; during rest, it slows down. The body makes all these heart rate adjustments automatically without a person even being aware of them.

God made the heart to function perfectly for a lifetime. God's children need to co-operate with the Creator so that this marvelous heart machine can continue to sustain the life of God's creation. To do this, we must live God's health plan: specifically for the heart, this includes exercising and eating whole foods. It also means avoiding caffeine, smoking, and other things that over-stimulate or damage the heart. We honor God by exercising moderation in things that are good and abstaining from things that are harmful to our bodies.

The vascular system houses the rushing river of life - His blood. The Bible tells us "the life of the flesh is in the blood". (Leviticus 17:11) Did you know that the average adult body has approximately 10 pints of life-imparting blood? This river of life flows constantly, taking fresh supplies of oxygen and nutrients to all of the millions of cells in the body and removing carbon dioxide and other waste products. It is very hard to imagine how complex the blood actually is.

The blood contains three types of cells: red blood cells, white blood cells, and platelets. The most numerous are the red blood cells. There are about a billion red blood cells in just a few drops of blood. Red blood cells get their red color from an iron-containing pigment called *heme*. Heme, combined with a particular protein, forms hemoglobin. This remarkable molecule has the ability to bind with oxygen or carbon dioxide and carry it through the blood. The life span of the red blood cell is only about three months, but in that short amount of time, it passes through the heart and the entire circulatory system about 1.3 million times.

White blood cells are less numerous than red blood cells; one drop of blood contains several thousand white blood cells. However, although fewer in number, they are equally as important as red blood cells. Without white blood cells, you could not survive for long because their job is to fight disease-causing bacteria or viruses that enter the body. There are five basic types of white blood cells, each of which was created to do a specific job in protecting the body. They search out foreign cells like an army of defending soldiers by traveling through the tissues and blood. When a white blood cell finds a foreign, disease-producing cell, it brings the foreign cell inside itself (a process known as phagocytosis) and then uses chemicals to destroy it.

The white blood cell that purifies the body from disease can be thought of as a replica of the earthly temple mentioned in the Old Testament (Exodus 25:8-9) where men came to be purified from their sins. Foreign invader cells that threaten the physical life of the body are similar to the impurities of sin that threaten the spiritual life of the body. In the body, the cell membrane that surrounds a white blood cell corresponds to the outer fabric curtain that surrounded the courtyard of the earthly temple. In the body, a foreign, disease-causing cell is brought through the cell membrane into the open inner area (cytoplasm) within the white blood cell. In a similar way, a sinful person went through the outer fabric curtain and into the courtyard of the earthly temple, bringing an animal with him to sacrifice as payment for his disease of sin. In the body, the foreign, disease-causing cell is killed and dissolved by cellular enzymes released by a lysosome. In a similar way, the animal representing sin was killed and burned at the courtyard altar by fire kindled by the priest. Another part of the white blood cell is the endoplasmic reticulum that surrounds the nucleus and produces carbohydrates, lipids (oils and fats), and proteins (the building blocks of life). In a similar way, the next structure in the earthly temple was the holy place. It contained a table with loaves of bread (carbohydrates), representing all of the tribes of Israel; a golden lampstand filled with oil and continually burning to represent the presence of the Holy Spirit; and the altar of incense, where incense and prayers were mingled to build a relationship with God. The most important part of the white blood cell is the nucleus where the DNA is located. DNA directs and commands all of the activities of the cell. In a similar way, the most holy place of the earthly temple contained the presence and throne of God (the mercy seat) above the ark that contained the Ten Commandments of God that were to direct all the activities of men. The Bible says "Know ye not that your body is the temple of the Holy Spirit who is in you, whom you have from God and that you are not your own. For you have been bought with a price; therefore, glorify God in your body and in your spirit, which are God's" (1 Corinthians 6:19-20). In a small way, God has placed important spiritual information that he wants us to remember in this miniature representation within a white blood cell.

The lung is another vital organ. In an adult, each lung weighs only one pound and is largely filled with air, and yet it performs one of the most important functions in the body. The average person breathes over 23,000 times each day. That adds up to 300 million breaths that inhale 75 million gallons of air in a lifetime. The lungs themselves do not have muscles; instead, when a person breathes, the diaphragm and muscles between the ribs contract to expand the chest cavity. This, in turn, creates a vacuum that causes the lungs to expand and draw in air through the nose and/or mouth. The air rushes through millions of tiny air passages only .01 of an inch in diameter into microscopic air sacs. Each air sac is covered with a network of tiny capillaries, very, very small blood vessels that only allow one red blood cell at a time to pass through them. As each red blood cell passes through, it releases the waste product carbon dioxide (which is then exhaled by the lungs) and picks up life-sustaining oxygen from the fresh air in the lungs. It is very important that the lungs be kept clean and healthy. The Creator built into the respiratory system tiny pollution trappers called cilia. These hairs are so tiny that they can only be seen with a microscope, and yet tens of millions of them are working in the air passageways with each breath. The cilia move in waves, beating twelve times a second to push captured dirt and dust up and out of the lungs.

Like the heart, the lungs work automatically without any conscious control. Although we can voluntarily make ourselves take a breath at a particular time, it is a good thing that the Creator designed the respiratory system with a primarily automatic function. If we had to think about each breath, there would be little time left to think about anything else!

God made the lungs to function perfectly for a lifetime. When we cooperate with God, we will recognize the importance of deep, cleansing breathing, fresh air, exercise, and avoidance of dust, chemicals, and pollutants in the air we breathe. Without deep breathing, the lungs lose some of their capacity for oxygen exchange. Most people know about the link between cigarette smoking and/or breathing secondhand smoke and lung cancer, but they do not know that smoke paralyzes the cilia that clean the air flowing to the lungs. When a person smokes, even for two weeks, those tiny pollution trappers begin to die, and this allows dust and dirt to enter the lungs. Healthy lungs are a bright pink color. The lungs of people who smoke become dark and gray from accumulated dirt and pollution. However, if a smoker quits smoking, the lungs will rebuild, and the cilia will start working again! Truly, our bodies are "fearfully and wonderfully made" by our great Creator!

Consider the construction and function of the largest organ of the body, the skin. The skin wraps the adult body in about twenty square feet of a tough, yet delicate tissue that weighs about seven pounds. The skin contains millions upon millions of microscopic oil glands, sweat glands, and hairs. The skin waterproofs the body and prevents the entrance of bacteria and viruses as well as harmful substances from the outside world. Skin keeps the "inside" enclosed and protected. The skin also contains nerve endings that whisk electrical messages of touch, temperature, or pain to the brain. Sunshine striking the skin creates the body's own natural source of vitamin D. The skin also helps regulate the body's temperature. When a person becomes too hot, tiny blood vessels in the skin open up to radiate heat away from the body. When the body becomes cold, these blood vessels narrow to help the body keep heat in. The skin is continually renewing itself and casting off dead cells; this helps prevent pathogens from gaining entrance. The skin is the body's "first line of defense" against injury and disease. The skin could be called an amazing envelope that protects the other amazing systems that exist within the human body. God is so intimately acquainted with every part of our bodies that the Bible even declares, "Indeed, the very hairs of your head are all numbered." (Luke 12:7)

Have you ever thought about where you came from and where and how your life began? All men, women, and children contemplate this question sometime during their lifetimes. Many of us believe that God created us, but can we understand how He did it? Probably not! No man can fully understand how God creates. Even with our finite intelligence, let us contemplate some of these questions.

After a spermatozoon from the father and an ovum from the mother unite, the phenomenon of life begins. Everyone starts out as this single cell. That one cell contains DNA that has the blueprint of what the entire body will be like, everything from a person's gender to the color of the eyes and hair, and right on down to molecules in the tissues and enzymes. The original cell becomes two cells, then four. The four become eight, the eight become sixteen, the sixteen become thirty-two. On and on these cells continue to multiply at an amazing rate of speed. The body contains approximately 100,000,000,000 (one hundred trillion), each containing its own DNA blueprint. The fact that these cells all work in harmony, each doing their own appointed work, is amazing! But even more amazing is the fact that the Bible declares that God knew each of us even *before* we were conceived! "Now the word of the Lord came to me saying, "Before I formed you in the womb, I knew you."" (Jeremiah 1:4-5)

In adulthood, new cell growth continues, but only for the replacement of existing cells that die. Accelerated rates of cell growth are only seen in disease cells. In an adult, over the course of a year, practically every cell in the body is replaced. Scientists have confirmed that 98 percent of the atoms in the body were not there a year ago. Think of that--a year from now, every one of us will have, in a manner of speaking, a new body. If each cell's needs are properly met, it will live healthfully and function properly, reproducing and replacing itself with another new, healthy, and strong cell.

Unfortunately, as the aging process progresses, the new cells that take the place of dying cells are often of an inferior quality because, over time, cellular DNA is damaged by exposure to radiation, chemicals, and so forth.

This is not how God intended it to be. If we use the genealogy of Adam and his descendants as found in the Bible, we can determine that Adam lived to be 930 years old! Also, Adam's height was much greater than ours is today. Although we can no longer live that long, we can still honor our bodies and obey God's laws of health. We can still eat the original diet given to man, and that diet has demonstrated to be very effective in improving the quality and length of life.

SUMMARY AND CONCLUSIONS

Our Creator made the human body to work as one of the most complex and wonderful things of His creation. Each system works together to make the body function. Nothing that man has ever made can duplicate God's masterpiece - the human body is fashioned in the image of God.

Yes, you are magnificent, created in the very image of God. Although generations of sin have marred our human bodies, it is still God's intention and plan to bring man back to the perfection he once had. This is begun on this earth by obedience to God's laws of health and is finalized for all eternity by the plan of salvation, which completely restores man and brings back the perfection in which he was first created.

Chapter Five
The Eight Laws of Health

God made earth inhabitable for men and animals. All living things have been given the ability to use natural resources, such as the atmosphere (fresh air), the sun, water, etc. Our planet was designed to sustain life and, if used properly, provide good health and a comfortable living for every creature. God gave us natural laws so that we could lead lives that are well balanced. Unfortunately, since leaving the Garden of Eden, mankind has been making his own laws, regarding not only religion, but also regarding the care of his body.

God designed laws in this universe for everything that we do. The author of our moral laws is also the author of the natural laws. If we do not obey these laws, we must suffer the consequences! If we want *good* health, then we must put into practice all eight of these natural laws.

1. Pure Air is Essential for Radiant Health

Air is the most important nutrient. This is obvious because as little as three minutes of deprivation will have very apparent and serious effects not only on our health but also on our very existence.

Pure air is the first essential of a healthy body. We can live without eating food for several weeks and without water for several days, but we cannot live without air. Air is so necessary that we cannot even commit suicide by just stopping breathing. If we hold our breath to the point of blacking out, our brainstem automatically takes over and causes us to start breathing again.

One of the important functions of air is to provide oxygen for the combustion (metabolism) of ingested nutrients. Without adequate oxygen, each cell cannot complete its functions. Without adequate oxygen, the cells and organs that eliminate the waste products of metabolism cannot function effectively. When the supply of oxygen is diminished, waste and poisons can accumulate. Any health treatment that does not encourage the use of good, clean, and fresh air will be significantly compromised in its effectiveness.

Pure, natural air a gift from God. The rays of the sun sterilize it. Rainwater washes and cleanses it. It is purified by the synergistic action of plant life. Plants use our exhaled carbon dioxide and, in exchange, provide us with fresh supplies of life-giving oxygen. With the disappearance of many of our forests and the effects of industrially generated pollutants, the supply of fresh, pure air is almost nonexistent in our day-to-day living and working environments. Instead of life-giving oxygen in abundance, there is an abundance of carbon dioxide, carbon monoxide, and other pollutants from tobacco smoke, automobile emissions, industrial wastes, burning vegetation, and so forth.

Pure, fresh air oxygenates and enlivens the body. Impure air is one of the greatest causes of poor health. Health-conscious people should be knowledgeable about their environments and the quality of the air they breathe. Air quality tends to be best at early morning and late evening. The best supply of clean, fresh air can be found in the mountains, in large wooded areas, near large bodies of water and in some remote places far from industry and automobiles. Clean, fresh air is negatively charged, and polluted air is positively charged. In instances where indoor air is poor, a negative ion generator can be used to improve air quality. There is no real substitute, however, for fresh, clean outdoor air. Because fresh air is so important to health, we need to make an effort to breathe natural clean air, for example, during outdoor morning exercise. This will impart to us a vitality that is superior and cannot be matched by breathing stale, re-circulated air or that found in smoky rooms, congested offices, or noisy factories.

The effects of poor air quality are well known. Cigarette smoking is linked to emphysema and lung cancer, and even second-hand smoke is linked to sudden infant death syndrome (SIDS) in babies. Discomfort and symptoms related to office environments have led to such phrases as *sick-building syndrome*. This is particularly noted in sealed buildings with centrally controlled, mechanical ventilation. Associated conditions include allergies, infections, Legionnaire's disease, and worsening of asthma because of air-borne irritants.

SOME IMPORTANT QUALITIES OF AIR

1. Air is an *essential* food. In fact, it contributes more to health and vitality than any other edible food and must be present for the performance of many vital functions. The oxygen in air is carried by the blood to every cell in the body and is essential for cellular metabolism.
2. Air contains electricity. Fresh air charges your nerves and muscles with electricity and increases your energy.
3. Air is a healing agent. A wound will not heal without air. It acts as both a purifier and a deodorizer.
4. Fresh air acts as an agent in producing a more positive mental attitude. It strengthens and nourishes the nervous system. Foul air is depressing and stressful for your body.
5. The oxygen in air is replenished by the leaves of trees. We, in turn, breathe out carbon dioxide, an essential nutrient for plants! God created this synergistic cycle so that we would always have fresh supplies of oxygen to maintain optimum health.

Daily exposure to fresh air is very important for vibrant health. Each day you should begin with an air bath. Exposing your body to the air with as little clothing as is practical can be very refreshing and revitalizing for your entire body.

Basic deep breathing can be incorporated into your daily routine. Most people tend to breathe significantly less than their true capacity. Deep breathing, which starts in the diaphragm, is extremely important to physical health.

The lung is a major organ of elimination. Shallow breathing limits the amount of carbon dioxide and other harmful gases that can be eliminated through your lungs. Breathing should be relaxed and done within your capacity. Breathing in (inhalation) energizes the body and breathing out (exhalation) relaxes the body. When using breathing exercises, it is important that your exhalation be at least as long as your inhalation, and most authorities recommend that exhalation be slightly longer than inhalation.

Most aerobic activities encourage deep breathing to promote functional integrity of the respiratory system. Certain disciplines like yoga, martial arts, and several holistic techniques encourage deep, controlled, and health-promoting breathing.

In summary, breathing is the simplest and most important bodily function we have for sustaining life. Deep breathing, exercise that promotes breathing, and breathing fresh, pure air are all ways that we can provide the oxygen that we need to promote radiant health.

2. PURE WATER IS ESSENTIAL FOR RADIANT HEALTH

The most precious of all liquids is water. We can live without water for perhaps a week or two at the most, and deficiencies in this area are very well understood and documented. Interestingly, our earth is 70 to 75 percent water, and our bodies are also 70 to 75 percent water, demonstrating the model of abundance and availability: what man needed most is what God created in abundance.

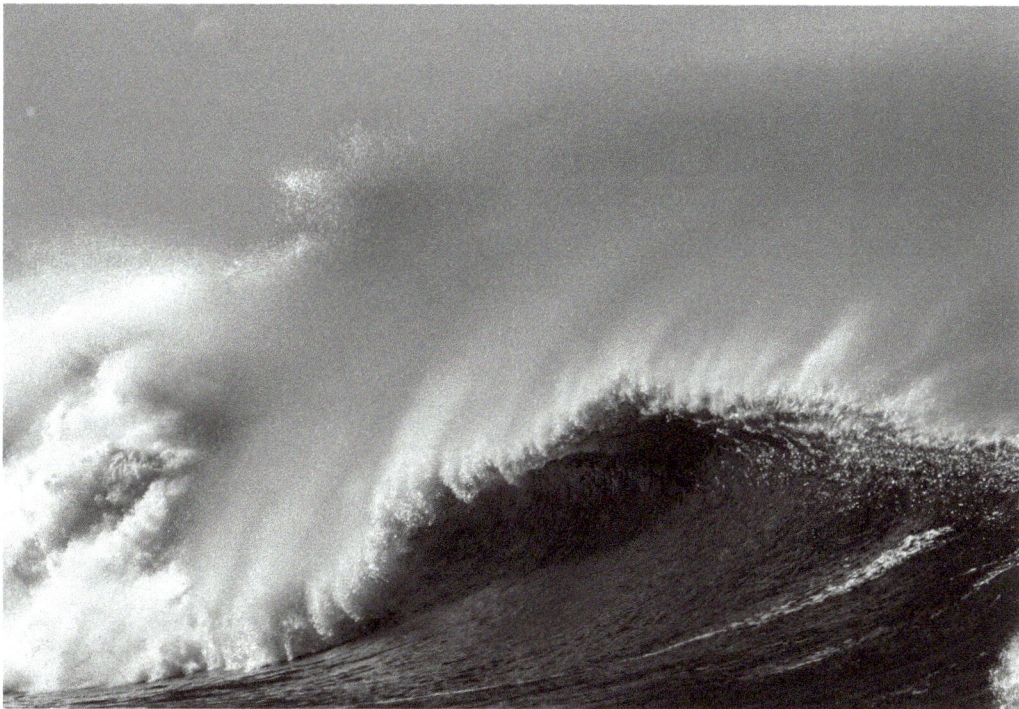

The planet is 70-75 percent water and so are our bodies
- we are an exact template of the planet.

The body of a 150-pound man contains approximately 105 pounds of water. Water is essential for the function of every cell of the body. Almost every cell and tissue of our body not only contains water and is continually bathed in fluid, but also requires water to perform its functions! The gray matter of the brain is approximately 85 percent water, the blood is approximately 83 percent water, and the muscles are approximately 75 percent water. All major processes in the body, including circulation, digestion, and elimination require the presence of water. Body temperature is regulated by the evaporation of water from the skin. Because water is so essential to every cell and every function of the body, the kidneys reabsorb and recycle water as much as possible. However, significant amounts of water are continuously being excreted to carry waste products in the urine, and so the body's supply of water must be constantly replenished.

Health conscious people should be knowledgeable about their environment and quality of the water they use. Water pollution abounds because of contamination by sewage pumped into rivers and oceans; runoff from garbage dumps; oil spills; industrial wastes such as mercury, lead, and polychlorinated bisphenols (PCBs); chemical fertilizers and pesticide residues; and so forth. Many of these substances are present in public drinking water because the law allows "acceptable levels." Mandated chlorination of public water adds yet another chemical. Distilled water is the best and purest type of water, but for those who only have access to tap water, water filtration systems or bottled water are often the most practical means of getting quality water. For most purposes, and especially for cleansing and fasting programs, distilled water provides the best results.

It is important to ensure adequate water intake to maintain bodily functions. A lack of the sensation of thirst is not always the best indicator of the body's need for water; some people do not feel thirsty until their bodies are quite dehydrated.

Your body requires approximately sixty-four to eighty ounces of water (eight to ten eight-ounce glasses) a day. A general rule is one ounce of water for every two pounds of body weight, modified to meet special circumstances such as activity level, outside temperature, and health status. This recommendation of eight to ten glasses a day is for a cooked-food-oriented diet. However, living a natural lifestyle and eating a natural diet consisting primarily of fruits and vegetables provides the body with a built-in supply of water. Since fruits and vegetables are high water-content foods (more than 70 percent water), less additional drinking water is required. Most animals in the wild live on fruits and vegetables and drink very modest amounts of water. In addition, the water contained in fruits and vegetables has been distilled by the synergistic action of the sun and provides pure, clean, thirst-quenching, and life-giving water. Eating an adequate amount of live, fresh fruits and vegetables gives the body an abundance of the purest naturally distilled water that is full of fragrance, organic minerals, and life-giving nutrients.

Altering the water content of foods by excessive cooking and processing compromises the quality of both the food and its water content. When unnatural, processed foods are taken into the body, nature tries to counteract them by diluting them. This in turn causes thirst. Satisfying this thirst with the introduction of large quantities of unnatural fluids can be very distressful and harmful to the optimum performance of our bodies. Over-consumption of fluid, even water, causes several problems, including bloating, excessive water retention, distention of blood vessels and organs and other harmful results. It can also overtax the kidneys and cause excessive urination.

When required, water is best taken between meals and should be sipped, not gulped down. It should be at room temperature or warmed for best results. Iced water, in particular, can be very harmful to the internal organs, especially the kidneys. It tends to shock and put the internal organs into spasm. Digestion is stopped until the water can be warmed to body temperature, thereby delaying or causing incomplete food breakdown.

Water is also beneficial externally. It can be used to reduce the heat of the body in cases of fever, increase the heat of the body in cases of low vitality, cleanse the skin, and tonify the body.

Hydrotherapy, properly administered colonics, contrast foot baths and showers and steam baths are some of the external uses of water that promote and maintain health. Hydrotherapy is the special therapy that uses the application of hot and cold water treatments. Colon hydrotherapy uses warm water to gently clean out and stimulate reflex points in the colon. Contrast showers and foot baths, which employ alternating hot and cold water, relax the muscles, improve the circulation, and strengthen the immune system. Steam baths open and cleanse the pores of the skin.

In summary, water is one of the simplest and most important substances we can use for sustaining our bodies. Water taken internally, particularly in the purified form found in fruits and vegetables, and water administered externally are both ways in which we can care for our bodies and promote radiant health.

3. SUNLIGHT IS ESSENTIAL FOR RADIANT HEALTH

We can live without sunlight for extended periods of time, longer than without air or water, but not without serious consequences. All life on earth depends on the energy of the sun. In short, all life on earth, including human beings, would cease to exist if there was no sunshine. Sunshine helps maintain the ambient temperatures of the earth. In this way it supports both plant and animal existence and is a vital ingredient in our environment.

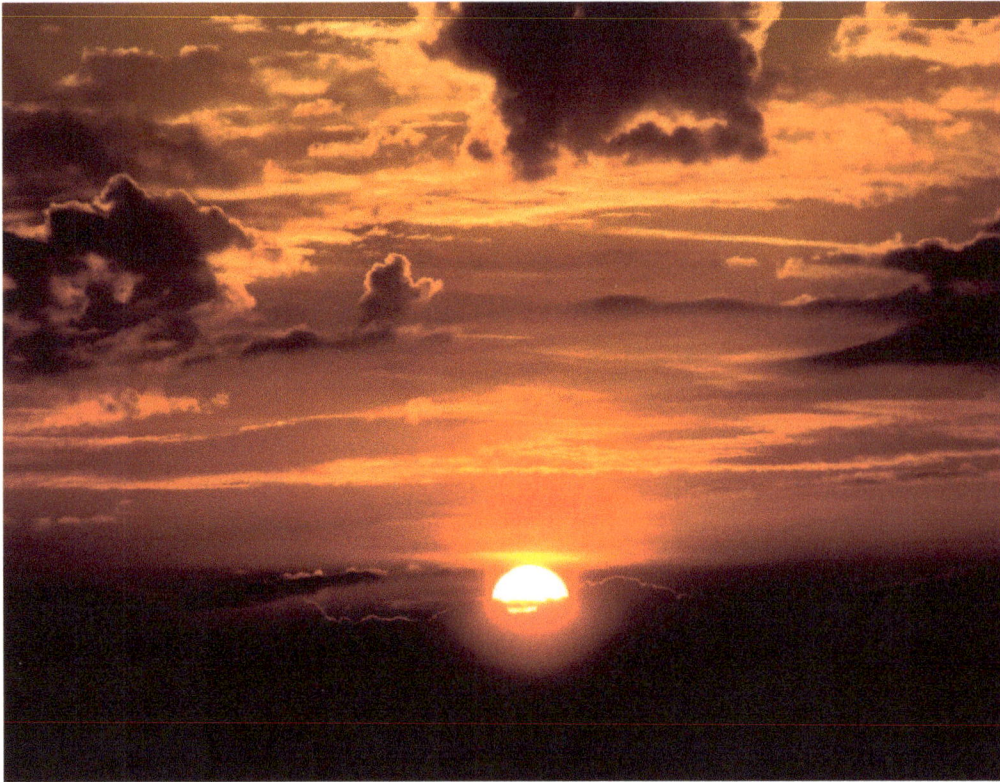

Sunlight is composed of many different energy levels, transmitted in the form of electromagnetic waves. The rays of the sun expose the body to three different wavelengths of light:

1. Invisible light: The invisible light generated by the sun includes both ultraviolet and infrared light. Ultraviolet light (5 percent of solar radiation) provides the majority of the biological effects, both positive and negative, to the body. Infrared light (54 percent of solar emissions) provides warmth.
2. Visible light: This comprises 40 percent of the solar radiation.
3. Other types of waves: The shorter waves consist of cosmic rays, gamma rays, and x-rays. The longer waves are radio and electromagnetic waves.

Some of the obvious benefits of the sun are the production of vitamin D in the skin, improved vitamin and mineral absorption, particularly calcium, and overall improvement in metabolic function and efficiency. In addition to the known nutrient-giving properties of the sun, there are many complex and even unknown benefits. As a secondary benefit, the abundant energy and life-giving properties that sunlight gives to the plant kingdom have similar positive effects on humans who eat those plants. The full-spectrum light and energy provided by the sun supplies the subtle, vibratory energy underlying all plant and human function. Exposure to the sun results in a healthy-looking complexion, energized blood, and overall good health. In contrast, insufficient sunlight results in a pale complexion, lowered physical vitality, and poor health.

Some of the important effects of the sun on your body are as follows:

1. Chemical. It unlocks the vitamins in your food. The process of digestion is incomplete without sunshine. The more light and heat we receive from the sun, the less heavy food we require. Sunlight in effect controls the chemistry of the blood.

2. Physical. Sunlight warms your body and at the same time energizes it. Sunshine helps and encourages every important function of the body. When sun shines on your skin it quickly stores up a tremendous amount of energy in your body. The nerve endings absorb the vibrant energy and transmit this energy to your entire nervous system. Natural sunlight contains the full spectrum of colors, which provides the best medium for visual acuity. The underlying energy systems of your body are constantly feeding on and storing up the life-giving elements from the rays of the sun. Sunshine, like air, acts as a stimulant, tonic, and healer. Some bacteria cannot live in direct sunlight, and many diseases are curable by allowing the sun to come in direct contact with the diseased part of the body for various periods of time. Sunshine is both a natural and effective healing agent. Eating in sunlight, when practical, enhances digestion and encourages a natural diet. A healthy, natural diet, in turn, enhances interest in and tolerance of sunlight. If your body has the right nutrients, it will respond very favorably to sunlight.

3. Psychological. Exposure to sunshine offers the experience of peace, joy, happiness, and a feeling of relief and freedom. The mind immediately senses that the body is in its natural medium, and the thoughts begin to take on a loftier aspect.

In modern times, we noticed a decline in the interest in sunshine. Up until a few years ago, the marvelous, health-giving power of sunlight was practically ignored by the general public and was familiar to only a handful of people. Now there seems to be an awakening to the wonderful beneficial effects of the sun's rays for the health and vitality of the human body and the ill effects that are caused by a lack of sunlight. Psychologically, lack of sufficient sunlight has been linked to seasonal affective disorder (SAD), a mood disorder of depression that appears during the winter months when there is less sunlight. On the other hand, overexposure to sunlight should be avoided at all times, especially exposure to midday sun in the summer months. As in many areas of life, moderation in those things that are healthful and abstinence from all things that are harmful is a valuable principle that applies to sunlight.

In summary, sunlight is one of the simplest and most important substances we can use for sustaining our bodies. Sunshine is free and its rays invigorate the body in many ways that promote radiant health.

4. Good Nutrition is Essential for Radiant Health

God made our bodies and our minds. He also provided us with a set of health laws for the ongoing maintenance of our bodies. If we eat the foods God intended us to use in the way God intended us to use them, then we will have good, strong, healthy bodies. If we don't follow these dietary rules, then our bodies will suffer as a result and eventually become diseased.

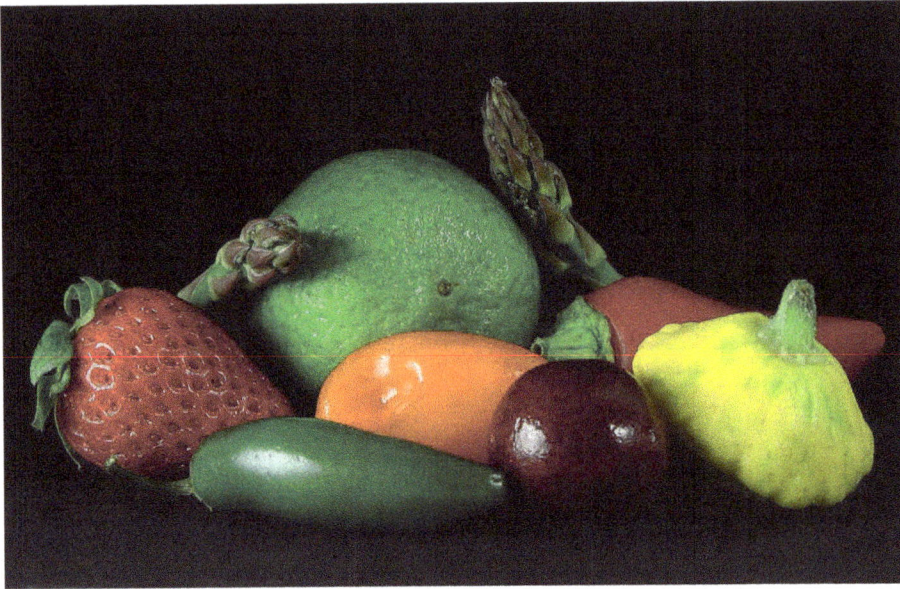

Fundamentally, the best foods for physical nourishment and health are living, whole foods as they were created by God and provided by nature. All the knowledge we have gained since the beginning of time continually supports this simple fact. Nature, in the form of plant foods, supplies all the food and medicine we need for physical health. Nature provides the most perfect food laboratory - one that yields an abundant menu of wholesome vitamins, minerals, proteins, carbohydrates, fats and other essential known and unknown nutrients. Fruits, vegetables, nuts, grains, seeds and edible herbs, properly prepared and in adequate amounts, supply all the nutrients required for developing and maintaining optimum health. Especially when eaten raw, the life of the food in the form of enzymes is still present and is highly beneficial to the body. This forms the basis of the dietary principles of original medicine.

In my book, *Basic Principles of Total Health*, I present a "hierarchy of nutrients" that ranks types of foods - from the best to the worst - as far as their ability to promote optimum, radiant health. This hierarchy is an alternative to the popular food pyramid, and it provides a perspective on nutrition that is in harmony with the original medicine concepts and principles.

The meaning of proper diet goes beyond eating a variety of healthy foods. It also includes eating those foods in the proper quantities and at the right time of the day. At one time, people grew and ate their own (native) simple foods, depending upon where they lived. Today the world has become so small due to rapid transportation that we now have food upon our tables from around the world any time we choose. In the sheer abundance of available foods, we have greater temptations today and greater opportunities to overeat. Indulgence of appetite and gluttony are prevalent and are ruinous to good health. Alcoholic and stimulating drinks consumed as companions to poor food choices further compromise our health. Not only is the correct quantity and quality of food important, but the time of food consumption must also be considered for maintaining good health. The breakfast meal should be the most nourishing meal of the day because it supplies the nutrients to carry us through the day. Instead, sugar-rich foods and coffee are commonly consumed as a breakfast. This causes a quick rise in blood sugar and then a later fall in blood sugar with a sudden hunger that prompts overeating. This can lead to poor eating habits like snacking and eating continually throughout the day and evening and thereby forcing our stomachs to work constantly digesting food hour after hour. The evening meal should be light so that the stomach is empty before retiring in the evening. Instead, in the evening, large, complex meals and extra helpings of dessert are often consumed. This causes the digestive system to work all night trying to digest the food. Like the body, the stomach, too, needs rest. Without rest, it becomes prone to disease.

But even with worldwide shipping and the availability of many new natural foods, we have ignored this source of health and continue to turn to manufactured foods that are high in sugar, high in fat, and low in nutrition. Instead of putting fruits, vegetables, nuts, grains, seeds, and edible herbs on our tables and enjoying these whole foods with their full complement of nutrients and healthful benefits, many may prefer to eat white bread, white sugar, saturated fats, and commercially prepared foods that have been stripped of many nutrients only to be artificially "enriched" with a few vitamins and minerals. In America, we have a whole new generation that has been brought up on junk-food meals consisting of hamburgers, colas, candy bars, fried foods, etc. This diet has not only formed bad nutritional habits, but it has taken away a liking and a taste for the natural foods that are so essential to the growth and health of the body. Consequently, we are experiencing a prevalent increase in diseases even among the very young. Pediatricians note an outbreak of diseases previously seen only in adults, such as diabetes, obesity and, more recently, kidney stones are all attributable to a poor diet in young people. Malnourished mothers, eating nutritionally poor diets, are producing babies with even more compromised health. With the diseased conditions present in the animal kingdom, eating a flesh diet is affecting our physical, mental, emotional, and moral life. It is almost impossible to live a patient, pure, healthful life while ingesting diseased animal products. These modern, and yet impoverished, eating habits have taken their toll on whole nations, and combating diseases caused by poor nutrition is now a way of life.

In summary, nutrition is an incredibly important factor in maintaining good health. Fruits, vegetables, grains, nuts, and herbs as whole foods are the most healthful. Commercially prepared foods have far fewer nutrients, and we compound this lack of nutrients by eating too much of the wrong foods at the wrong time. Unlike fresh air, fresh water, and sunshine, wholesome foods are not free, but God has given us the opportunity and the responsibility of using knowledge to make healthy food choices that invigorate the body and promote radiant health.

5. EXERCISE IS ESSENTIAL FOR RADIANT HEALTH

Exercise is another important support for the optimal performance of your body. It contributes to both the nourishment of your body and the elimination of waste. The fundamental principle of exercise as it relates to health is movement. Without movement, all life ceases to exist. In death all systems of your body - including the heart, brain, and circulatory system - stop "moving." If anything in the universe stops moving, its function is altered. This underlying principle of movement is the factor that promotes and supports optimal health. Movement engages all the major systems in your body, including the muscular, skeletal, nervous, endocrine (glands), and lymphatic systems.

In general, most people tend to use only about 50 of the more than 600 muscles in their bodies. This often results in overuse of less than 10 percent of our muscles with relatively inactivity of the rest, and this can result in several disease processes. Using a variety of individualized exercises or movements (based on genetic or environmental conditions) offers many advantages to optimizing health and wellness.

Anything that encourages the natural movement of the body contributes to health. The type and amount of exercise you choose are subject to the same rules of temperance and balance as the foods you eat. Whether walking; running; swimming; doing aerobics, yoga, tai chi, or martial arts; weightlifting; gardening; or pursuing any other activity, the following principles contribute to a healthy approach to exercise. All exercise should

- be enjoyable and relaxing
- be free of strain and pain
- use as many muscles and joints as is feasible
- use a variety of movements
- balance strength with flexibility and stretching
- cause you to breathe deeply
- ensure adequate rest.

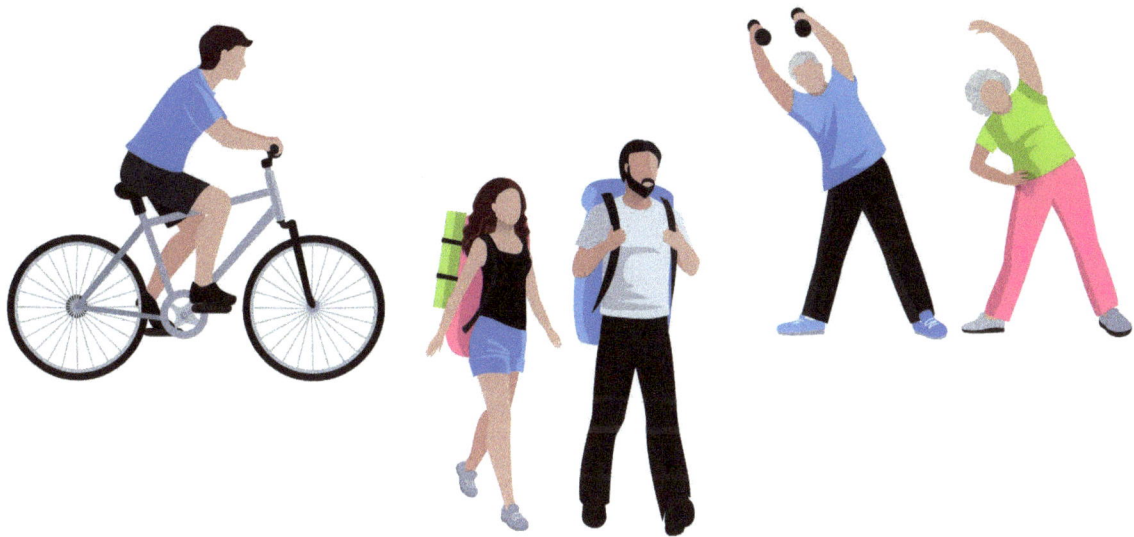

SOME IMPORTANT BENEFITS OF EXERCISE

Regular exercise is not only a preventive measure; it also works to maintain health at its best. There are many benefits of physical exercise. Some of them include the following.

- Exercise makes one more energetic and gives a sense of well-being.
- Exercise helps to lower high blood pressure. The *New England Journal of Medicine* published a study that found that aerobic exercise significantly lowered blood pressure in patients with hypertension.
- Exercise strengthens bones. Research conducted at Washington University School of Medicine in St. Louis demonstrated that a woman can increase her bone mass by 2 to 3 percent per year (for as long as the study was conducted) by doing weight-bearing exercises.
- Exercise promotes an increase in HDL cholesterol (good cholesterol). A study of nearly 3,000 men revealed that exercise was associated with higher HDL levels.
- Exercise helps in the management of diabetes. Harvard researchers documented that exercise decreases the risk of developing diabetes in adulthood. Exercise increases the ability of cell membranes to transport glucose into muscle cells. This particular transportation is not dependent on insulin, thus lowering the insulin requirement.
- Exercise improves communication in those with Alzheimer's disease. In a study examining communication skills of two groups of Alzheimer's patients, more than 40 percent of the group in a walking exercise program experienced significant improvement in communication skills, whereas the group who were given conversation lessons experienced no significant improvement.

- Exercise improves mental health. A study of patients not suffering from Alzheimer's disease showed measurable improvement in memory after an aerobic exercise program of nine to ten weeks' duration. With increased activity, older people showed improved mental function. There was a clear linear relationship between the level of activity and the level of mental ability. Through regular, active use of the body, one can discover a greater sense of well-being, far greater vitality, and a calmer, more relaxed attitude toward daily pressures.
- Exercise improves cardiac function. It strengthens the heart, making it more efficient, so that it can pump a greater volume of blood with each contraction.
- Exercise improves quality of life. A consensus panel convened by the National Institute of Health identified other important benefits in quality of life from exercise such as better mental health, decreased stress, decreased anxiety and depression, and decreased risk of certain cancers.

In 1998 the *Oregonian* published a story about an elderly man, Ben Levinson, 103 years old, to be precise, who set a world record for the shot-put for men over 100. He threw the ball 10 feet and 1.25 inches. But for Ben the achievement was to be throwing at all, at over 100 years! Thirteen years before, Ben Levinson was a depressed, unfit 90-year-old, shuffling around, frail and obviously ready for the grave. Ben had become dependent and weak through lack of exercise. Fortunately for Ben, he met Dave Crawley, an athletics trainer, who challenged him to feel eighty again. Ben began a training program, walking 20 minutes a day at 2.5 miles per hour, and weight-training three or four times a week. "He's grown 2 inches just with better posture and more confidence," says Crawley.

If a fitness program could do that for this 90-year-old, just think what it could do for you!

In summary, exercise is an incredibly important factor in maintaining good health. The wonderful thing about exercise is that you can begin reaping its rewards regardless of how old you are when you begin. Again, God has given us the opportunity and the responsibility of using knowledge to make healthful choices that invigorate the body and promote radiant health.

6. Adequate Rest is Essential for Radiant Health

Adequate rest is imperative for optimum health. Rest brings restoration and replenishes the resources we use. Without rest, the body process of catabolism (breaking down) overrides that of anabolism (building up), resulting in disease and compromised health.

Sleep is the most important medium for rest. Short naps, peaceful and relaxing environments, mental quietness, and the avoidance of stress also contribute to rest for your body.

Given the fact that, in one day, the heart beats over 100,000 times, pumping blood through miles of blood vessels, we speak thousands of words, breathe 23,000 times, move major muscles hundreds of times, and operate some fifteen to twenty billion brain cells, no wonder sleep is important in restoring our energy and maintaining health. As Shakespeare wrote: "Sleep wraps up the raveled sleeve of care."

A newborn baby sleeps an average of twenty hours a day, a 6-year-old sleeps about ten hours, a 12-year-old sleeps about nine hours, and an adult sleeps approximately eight hours. Whether these averages are optimal varies, depending upon the individual. Breslow and Belloc in their famous Alameda County study showed that persons obtaining eight to nine hours of sleep per night seemed to have better health outcomes than did those sleeping shorter or longer periods of time. Occasionally there are individuals, such as Ben Franklin and Thomas Edison, who can get by with four or five hours of sleep a night, but these individuals are the exceptions rather than the rule. Many who only sleep for short periods of time at night also take short catnaps throughout the day. Albert Einstein required at least nine hours of sleep. Adequate sleep should prevent sleepiness and drowsiness during the day and promote a sense of well-being and alertness.

Students who study all night prior to an examination often suffer the consequences of sleep deprivation manifested in inferior grades. Work schedules that do not permit adequate sleep may result in increased inattention in the workplace and accidents and errors.

According to sleep experts, we go through various stages and certain cycles when we sleep. Each cycle lasts approximately ninety minutes. We start with stage one sleep, which is the lightest stage, and then progress to a deeper, stage two sleep. Stage three sleep is related to delta wave brain activity, which is the slowest and most relaxed brain wave activity. Stage four is our deepest stage of sleep. The most powerful healing and rebuilding take place during the fourth stage of sleep, which lasts approximately twenty to forty-five minutes. Then we gradually return through stage three, stage two, and stage one sleep. A complete and uninterrupted cycling through these stages allows us to awaken refreshed without an alarm clock, and this significantly contributes to optimal health.

In cases of compromised health or excessive physical and mental activity, rest is imperative for restoring and supporting your body's natural healing ability. It is the most important factor for replenishing spent resources.

Sleep patterns also influence the secretion of these hormones:

1. Cortisol. This hormone is secreted during the second half of the sleep period. It prepares the body for the activity of the next day. Cortisol has numerous effects, influencing blood glucose levels, regulating sodium and potassium concentrations, regulating blood pressure, and influencing muscle strength. One of its most important actions is its anti-inflammatory effect. Regular sleep habits result in regular patterns of cortisol secretion.
2. Growth hormone. This hormone is secreted at its maximal rate during sleep. Its hormone affects glucose and amino acid metabolism.
3. Melatonin. Secretion rates increase during the night but may have more of a role to play in sexual regulation than anything to do with sleep regulation.

There are several other factors that can have a positive or negative influence on sleep. These include the following:

- Regular exercise and the avoidance of excessive fatigue during the day are conducive to good sleep at night.
- The last meal of the day should be a light one taken a few hours prior to retiring. However, it should be skipped or consist of something light, like fruit, if sufficient time is not available for the stomach to digest the food before retiring.
- The stomach should not be full before going to sleep, as the stomach needs to be resting along with other parts of the body. The digestive system tends to use more energy than any other major system of the body, including the circulatory, respiratory, and nervous system. Therapeutic fasting provides another energy-conserving and resting opportunity for your body.
- Avoidance of alcohol, tobacco, caffeine, and other chemical substances that interfere with normal sleep patterns is advised.
- The time preceding retiring should be free of arguments, exciting TV, and stressful events. It should be a quiet time to wind down the day's activity and prepare for rest.
- A warm, not hot, bath may help relaxation before going to bed. Use the many relaxation techniques, including massage, meditation,8 and prayer to provide valuable rest that contributes to health and wellness. In addition to natural sleep and temperance in diet and lifestyle, relaxation techniques contribute to vibrant energy and optimum health.
- Irregularity in rising and going to bed, shift work, travel across time zones, and weekend changes in sleep all militate against good sleep patterns.
- A quiet bedroom, free of bright light and noise, properly ventilated, and of a comfortable temperature aid in sleeping.
- Medical conditions such as sleep apnea, respiratory disorders, cardiac conditions, phobias, and other psychiatric disorders may require professional assistance.

When God created the earth, He created night as a period of daily rest for both man and animals. The Lord our Creator knows that our bodies need a balanced daily rest -physically, mentally, emotionally, and socially. At the close of the creation week, God Himself "rested" on the seventh day as an example to man of how to rest from his labors each week because He also knows that in order to function optimally, we also need a weekly rest. Not only did God "rest", but He also blessed this day. "Remember the Sabbath day, to keep it holy. Six days you shall labor and do all your work: but the seventh day is the Sabbath of the Lord your God: in it you shall do no work: you, nor your son, nor your daughter, nor your manservant, nor your maidservant, nor your cattle, nor your stranger who is within your gates." (Exodus 20:8-10) NKJV

Rest at the appropriate times is beneficial and contains a blessing. The Bible says that there should be daily rest as well as a weekly rest, and even modern man has found that just such a rest meets all his needs by providing a much-needed break from the demands of the work. In addition, the Sabbath provides a special blessing not only of rest but also of fellowship. The Lord wants us to have fellowship with Him especially on the Sabbath day, for He created us as His children. Part of the blessing of the Sabbath rest comes as we support and relate to each other. Service to others provides a powerful rest from the self-focused and egocentric activities that often encumber us. "The Sabbath was made for man not man for the Sabbath"! Mark 2:27 NKJV Regular sleep and weekly rest empowers us to be receptive to the blessing of God so that He can fill our lives with His many blessings!

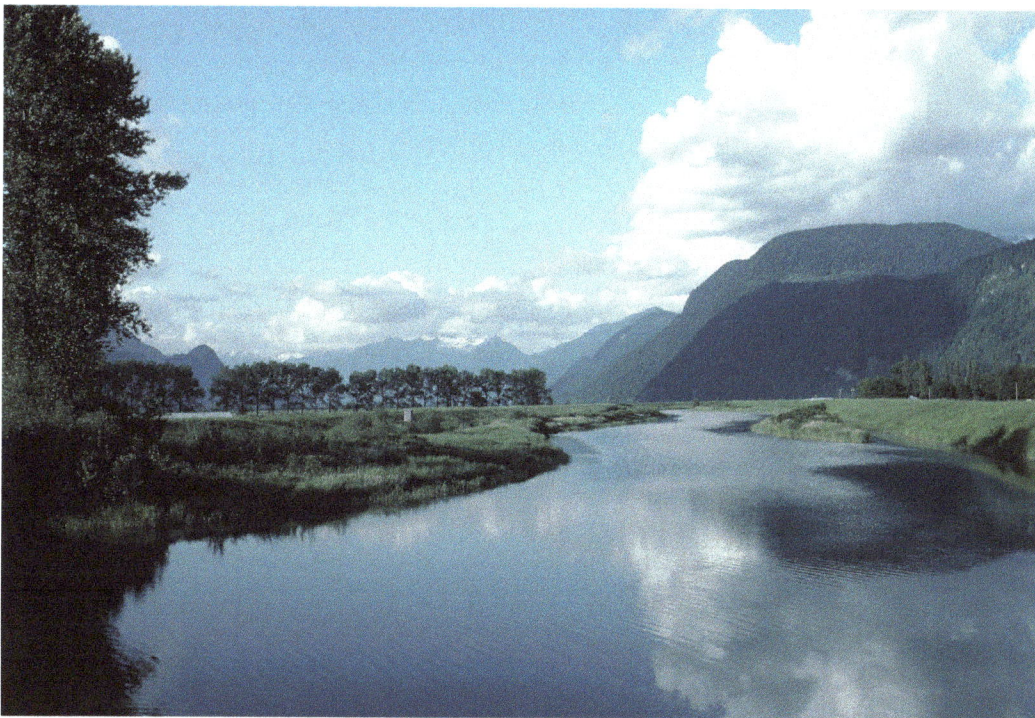

Even during periods of greatest stress and activity with deadlines, rest is essential. During World War II, increased productivity was achieved, not by a continuous, non-stop work schedule to increase production as was first tried, but later by a 48-hour work week. This demonstrated that, even under the pressures of war, people have limitations on their work capabilities and must rest if they are to do their best. On July 29, 1941, six months before the entry of the United States into the war, Prime Minister Winston Churchill announced in the House of Commons, "If we are to win this war it will be by staying power. For this reason, we must have one holiday per week and one week holiday per year". And this was voted into law!

Periodic rests include annual vacations. These vacations are not necessarily periods of inactivity, but of engagement in activities normally outside the scope of the daily routine. These times provide mental and emotional restitution and help to stimulate creativity and strengthen family relationships.

In summary, rest is an incredibly important factor in maintaining good health. The wonderful thing about rest is God has provided times of rest throughout the week—nightly rest for sleep and a weekly Sabbath rest to fellowship with Him and rest from our labors. Again, God has given us the opportunity and the responsibility of using knowledge to make healthful choices to rest the body and promote radiant health.

7. TEMPERANCE IS ESSENTIAL FOR RADIANT HEALTH

Temperance means to be moderate or sparing, using self-restraint and self-control. Moderation has a similar meaning. So when we speak of temperance, we are speaking of self-control. Another definition is "Moderation in those things that are healthful and abstinence from all things that are harmful."

Temperance and self-control are necessary to avoid health-destroying behaviors. Is there any sense in the moderate use of arsenic or strychnine? Definitely not! Everyone knows these are deadly poisons. However, some things, even things commonly used by many people - things like tobacco, alcohol, and addictive substances—are best totally avoided because of their poisonous effect on the body. Alcohol, tobacco, and other drugs are enticing because they are promoted as fun, stimulating, and as a release from stress and pain. Even many innocent-appearing popular beverages contain drugs. Theophylline lurks in tea, and caffeine is hidden in most coffee and colas. Fruit-flavored wine coolers contain alcohol. Using alcohol, tobacco, and other drugs in any amount is hazardous because they often lead to addiction and harm. Even some prescription drugs can be addictive, and they must be used with great caution and only when necessary. Drugs destroy purity of mind when they cause addiction. Drugs destroy purity of soul when intoxication leads to abuse, inappropriate sex, or violent behavior. Drugs destroy purity of body when they cause disease and even death. Instead of artificial stimulants with a subsequent crash, get your highs from exercise and enjoying the beauty of God's created world. In place of chemical depressants and stimulants, get your relaxation from sunlight, water, and rest.

Temperance, moderation, and balance are principles that underlie all other health factors. Although moderation is usually associated with avoiding harmful things like processed foods, caffeine, nicotine, alcohol, drugs, and other waste elements, it also includes the wise and judicious use of things that are good. Overeating and poor combinations of good food, over-supplementation with vitamins, indiscriminate use of herbs and other specialized products, and unbalanced amounts of exercise and rest can compromise optimum physical health. Moderation means using good common sense guided by the laws of health in God's word, the Bible. Moderation in diet is rewarded with mental and moral vigor. If moderation is not part of our everyday life, it is easier to succumb to the temptation of things that injure our health. Moderation provides the balance and self-control that permit the highest attainment of our physical, mental, and spiritual development.

In summary, temperance is an incredibly important factor in maintaining good health. Temperance means to abstain from everything that is harmful and to use judiciously that which is beneficial. Again, God has given us the opportunity and the responsibility of using knowledge to be temperate and make healthful choices that promote radiant health.

8. Trust in Divine Power Essential for Radiant Health

Of all the eight laws of natural health, this law should be the most sacredly cherished because our every breath, good health, and the essence of all healing come from the Creator.

All great civilizations have been founded on religious beliefs and moral values that lead to an orderly society. Belief in spiritual values is a strong motivator to treat others well and to develop peaceful human relationships. History demonstrates that faithless and amoral societies become so corrupt that they cannot survive. Belief is characteristic of science as well as religion. Just as faith in a scientific principle is verified when tests produce consistent results, so faith in God is validated when it brings consistent and satisfying results. Studies indicate that those with regular spiritual practices who meet with a faith community live longer, live better, and are far less likely to have a stroke or heart attack. Faith can empower you to overcome stress and destructive habits. Belief can give you peace of mind and enable you to reach your full potential through positive choices.

All of God's creation relies on God completely. The planets and their moons orbit in an orderly fashion through space, rotating at enormous speeds on their axis while racing along their lines of travel. The animals hunt their food, but it is God's hand that sends them their fare. "Consider the ravens, for they neither sow nor reap…yet God feeds them." (Luke 12:24). Even the flowers are under His care. "Consider the lilies, see how they grow; they neither toil nor spin, but even Solomon in all his glory could not clothe himself like one of these". (Luke 12:27). It is the human race alone that does not always recognize its total dependence on God's goodness and blessings. God made the world and all things in it, since He is Lord of heaven and earth…He Himself gives life and breath to all things…though He is not far from each one of us for in Him we live and move and have our being." (Acts 17:24-28)

Everyone needs to believe in something eternal and stable for viability and long-term health. Health at the spiritual level synergistically produces health at all levels in the mind and body. Your mind is energized with the vibrant health of positive thinking and emotions. Your body is ruled by the mind, and the body works to achieve Divine sustenance not just subsistence.

Challenges that we face at the physical or mental level can compromise our ability to focus on our spiritual growth and development. Like air, which is abundantly supplied and easily available, the spiritual element of our being is easy to take for granted and overlook, even though it so pervasively and abundantly provides for our life and well-being.

Spiritual realization is available to all who are seeking wisdom and truth. Many squander this powerful and abundantly provided path to total health, but the few who truly set aside some quiet time to embrace the perfect and mysterious aspect of the spirit, will find it. "Ask and it will be given to you, seek and you will find, knock at the door and it will be opened to you." (Matthew 7:7-9) When you hear the prompting of His spirit (God's voice speaking to you quietly), listen, and you will be rewarded with renewed health and wellness.

A spiritual life is available to all of us, regardless of our station in life or level of performance. This is the one aspect of our being in which we are all on a level playing field. It is the most powerful force of our being. An ounce of spiritual health can transcend pounds of physical and mental problems. Many mysterious and miraculous cures testify to this truly awesome phenomenon. Those who are wise enough to accept and capitalize on this aspect of their being can create the physiological and mental nutrients to overcome obstacles to achieving optimal health.

Spiritual growth and nourishment is a major aspect of all religions or philosophies. There are many paths that mankind has experienced during the quest for spiritual realization. Many sincere and well-intentioned religious organizations try to claim sole ownership of this realm, but the wisdom of men and institutions will always fall short of the enormous wisdom and power of the Creator of men.

Relying solely on human knowledge, science and its institutions will always compromise total health at all levels of our being, especially at the spiritual level. The mysteries which are still to be unraveled far outweigh the knowledge we have gained during our brief history here on earth. Spiritual health that is pure, peaceful, loving, and sincere is available to each of us.

While the spiritual part of our being is the most powerful aspect of human existence, it also tends to be both extremely complex and underutilized by many, and yet simply and powerfully utilized by some. What causes us to fall short of maximizing our spiritual support and nourishment? Don't we all want total health and happiness in our lives? The questions are easy, but the answers are not as simple. There are many distractions, including the daily activities of earning a livelihood, our natural pleasure-seeking ways, and so forth. At another level, our own pride, selfish motives, arrogant sense of self-worth, and refusal to accept truth can also act as stressful burdens that must be eliminated before we can experience true spiritual health.

Once we understand and appreciate our relative insignificance from a universal perspective and humbly submit to and accept the spiritual prompting of God as given to us through a pure and healthy mind, we begin the process of waste elimination that will eventually lead to spiritual growth. Regardless of our age, wealth, or wisdom, we are relatively powerless until we center our spiritual growth in an eternal God.

Spiritual health keeps our entire being in balance. It provides the healthy soil that brings forth good fruit. It prevents us from being overbearing. Just as fruit and vegetables are the staples for supporting our physical health, unconditional love and forgiveness are the primary staples for supporting spiritual health. Peace, joy, humility, and wisdom are the nuts, seeds, grains, and legumes that round out a complete whole-food diet that supports our spiritual health.

As we develop a relationship with our Creator, we experience a new and improved body, mind, and spirit. As we selflessly share our newfound pearls of health and vitality with our neighbors, we improve our own health, as well as that of our neighbors and our planet. The power of love, which is the life force of our spirit, creates, as it were, a new life and a new earth for us. Trusting in the Divine power that created us enables the harmonious integration of body, mind, and spirit. The earthly goal of physical health, which is temporal, is transcended to include spiritual health, which is eternal.

The following are health-promoting items that support an environment for optimal health at the spiritual level.

Acknowledgment of Our Dependence on a Higher Power

Human beings are subject to the higher laws of nature, just like all phenomena in the universe. Recognition of our human boundaries opens our body and mind to Divine healing forces. Acknowledgment of our dependence opens the pathway for us to achieve spiritual maturity.

It is fascinating when we stop to think about the awesome complexity and balance of the universe. The more we explore and learn, the greater our appreciation for how much more there is to know. By following the laws of nature and trusting in the Creator who governs our universe, health is enabled beyond today's limited comprehension.

Love for Our Fellow Man

Love's mysterious healing energy uplifts us personally and improves our social relationships. It is powerful enough to "heal" our entire planet.

Daily Exercise of Our Spiritual Self

Practice makes perfect. It is important to regularly spend some quiet time for the awakening of our inner mind and spiritual self. Daily Bible study, prayer, and service to others are among the most powerful spiritual calisthenics known to man. With the daily distractions of today's frenetic pace, daily focus on our spiritual side will guard our immune system against the ever-increasing health challenges we face.

Learning from Nature

Nature teaches many lessons regarding nurturing and healthy living. By observing, studying, and applying the powerful laws of nature to our lives, our spiritual enrichment overcomes the boundaries and mysteries of physical limitations.

An Active Prayer Life

Throughout history civilizations have demonstrated their natural propensity to communicate to a higher power. Prayer is legendary for its powerful healing influences. Throughout our recorded history and still today, it heals many conditions. There are many things that may seem right in the light of human knowledge that in the end lead to disappointing results. An active prayer life opens our minds and hearts to the Source of all knowledge, wisdom, and health.

Our spiritual nature is what differentiates us from every other living thing on our planet. Many of us instinctively feed ourselves with the healing energy assimilated through spiritual things. The spiritual element is the most powerful element of our being, one that allows us to transcend the limitations of all known human knowledge to receive a mysteriously perfect and lasting gift of health.

In my naturopathic practice, I like to start the personalized health plan for each client with the first and most important element. Namely, I instruct a client in this way: "Spend special time in prayer daily. God can do everything, and when we pray to Him, we can do everything He can do!"

Trust and reliance on a loving, powerful God give the ability to enjoy a healthful lifestyle. Complete belief in God permits Him to fill our lives with outrageous and radiant health!

SUMMARY AND CONCLUSIONS

The integrated and comprehensive use of the eight laws of health make up the most powerful, health-enhancing system known to man. These time-honored principles are the implementation of the original medicine concept. As important as nutrition or a proper diet is in relation to good health, it can be quite meaningless if we are not practicing all eight natural laws of health.

The effectiveness of all other methods of maintaining and enhancing health should be evaluated on the basis of their promotion of these foundational laws of health. We should be thankful for the power of these simple laws and apply them to ourselves and then lovingly share them with our family, friends, and associates, for a richer and healthier society, neighborhood, and world.

CHAPTER SIX
FINAL THOUGHTS ON ORIGINAL MEDICINE

Original medicine draws its knowledge and inspiration from the Bible with its descriptions of a Creator, the origin of man, and the original diet. Honor and glory belong to God alone for all health since He is the Originator and Creator of all things. All human beings and their inventions, systems, power, and wisdom are subordinate to His power and wisdom.

Original medicine embraces the fact that God is the Author of the natural laws of health and has placed within our power the means for obtaining knowledge of these laws of health. Original medicine encourages putting forth the needed effort to obtain knowledge of God's laws of life and the simple means He has chosen for the restoration of health. It is our duty to preserve our physical and mental powers in the best possible condition so that we may effectively serve our fellow man and Him. When sickness is the result of the transgression of natural law, we should seek to correct the error and then ask for the blessing of God. Those who refuse to improve the light and knowledge that have been mercifully placed within their reach are rejecting one of the means that God has granted them to promote spiritual as well as physical life.

The International Institute of Original Medicine (IIOM) Hierarchy of Healing includes the following original medicine principles:

1. Avoid all harmful factors causing or contributing to the condition.
2. Use natural, harmless, and simple remedies freely. These include air, water, sunlight, nutrition, exercise, rest, moderation, gratitude, benevolence, and trust in Divine Power.
3. Use "less harmful" remedies, such as selected natural substances and herbs, judiciously.
4. Only rarely, when all else has failed, turn to conventional drugs. Generally speaking, this should be as a last resort, not the first resort.
5. Pray, thanking God for His many blessings, and seeking His wisdom and guidance in all things including health and healing.

ORIGINAL MEDICINE AND NATUROPATHY

Original medicine presents its unique perspective within the more generalized health field known as naturopathy. Naturopathy emphasizes the curative powers of nature. Naturopathy also emphasizes the harmonious integration of body, mind, and spirit. Nutrition is an important factor in naturopathic healing. Naturopathy includes nourishing the body and eliminating waste from the body to improve the metabolic processes. Naturopathy strives to suspend or slow down the aging process. Disease is understood as a natural method of eliminating waste and correcting other ailments within the body. Naturopathy encourages and promotes personal responsibility, self-care, self-motivation, and education along with a more disciplined lifestyle that includes the basics of natural health care.

Naturopathic doctors work to restore and support the body's own healing ability using a variety of modalities including nutrition, herbal medicine, homeopathic medicine, oriental medicine, and therapeutic massage. The naturopath is a Doctor of Natural Healing and an expert on optimum lifestyle issues. The naturopath is able to educate and recommend a course of action that usually results in restoring a healthy, normal body and mind. Education, prevention, and a natural lifestyle are at the core of naturopathy.

The three basic principles of naturopathy are as follows.

1. The cause of disease is due to unnecessary wastes being accumulated in the body.
2. The body is always striving for the ultimate good of the individual. Naturopathy eaches how to listen to the body's signals.
3. Given the proper environment, the body has the power to heal itself and to return to its normal balance.

IIOM offers courses in original medicine as well as in naturopathy and natural ways of healing.

Original Medicine and Naturopathy Versus Allopathy

An important topic facing many students is the role of naturopathy as compared to the dominant infrastructure of allopathic medicine (also referred to as "conventional medicine").

Allopathic approaches tend to have the greatest applicability to acute health issues such as broken bones, severe bleeding, trauma, and advanced bacterial infections. They are not as effective for chronic, degenerative conditions resulting from compromised diet and lifestyle. Conversely, naturopathy tends to have its greatest applicability to chronic, degenerative conditions that result from compromised diet and lifestyle. Chronic degenerative conditions, such as cancer, diabetes, vascular diseases, AIDS, and so forth, comprise the overwhelming majority of health conditions - over eighty percent of health conditions as reported in various statistical charts and surveys.

For the benefit of our students, IIOM offers selected courses in "conventional medicine," such as anatomy and physiology, disease processes, and pharmacology. This integrated approach allows students to be knowledgeable about many aspects of conventional medicine. IIOM students who plan to open their own naturopathic practices particularly need to be aware of approaches used in conventional medicine when clients come to them seeking help.

Both approaches clearly have a place in today's health system where an integrated approach can many times be the most appropriate approach for certain conditions. However, the original medicine concept does not provide unqualified support for any particular system of health. It promotes any and all parts of various systems that are in harmony with Biblical themes and constructs for health of the total person - body, mind, and spirit. In any naturopathic or allopathic system, if the emphasis and credit is given to the healing power of men, institutions, herbs, drugs or other devices rather than to the Author and Creator of these things, then the original medicine view is that neither the naturopathic or the allopathic modality is right and appropriate. The original medicine is amenable to what can be called **Godopathy**, which acknowledges God as the wisdom, source, and power behind all true health and healing.

The foregoing chapters of this book were presented to lay the foundational principles of the concept of original medicine from the Bible and its teachings as embraced by the International Institute of Original Medicine. In the words of the inspired writer Ellen G. White, "There are many ways of practicing the healing arts, but there is only one that Heaven approves." Counsels on Diets and Foods, p. 301.2, Ellen Gould White Because the simplicity and validity of her writings on health and wellness offer excellent insights into Bible principles and have passed the test of time for generations, they have been quoted in this book and are presented in other IIOM courses as well.

The following excerpt from the writings of Ellen G. White is an excellent underpinning for the original medicine perspective on health and healing:

It is not safe to trust to physicians who have not the fear of God before them. Without the influence of divine grace, …the physician may claim to possess great wisdom and marvelous skill, while at the same time…his practice [is] contrary to the laws of health. Furthermore, the teaching of these physicians is continually leading away from the principles God has given us in regard to health, especially on the diet question. They say we are not living as we ought and prescribe changes that are contrary to the light God has sent, but the Lord our God assures us that He is waiting to be gracious; He invites us to call upon Him in the day of trouble. (Counsels On Health 456.2, 456.3)

We invite our students to weigh the practices, modalities, and benefits of original medicine, naturopathy, allopathy, and other health systems and draw their own conclusions.

Summary and Conclusions

There are many theories and teachings of health. The International Institute of Original Medicine (IIOM) offers a Biblical perspective to its valued students and encourages their personal study, reasoning, and verification in evaluating and adopting these principles for personal empowerment, physical, emotional, mental, and spiritual health.

IIOM courses provide materials from various sources that are in harmony with the original medicine concepts and principles. Our intent is to provide a template upon which any number of theories can be evaluated according to their consistency and harmony with the concepts and principles of the original medicine viewpoint. According to Proverbs 14:12 NKJV "There is a way that seems right to a man, but its end is the way of death". Our sincere hope is that our students will be equipped and empowered with time-tested health principles that have been proven to be the most powerful health-affirming system known to mankind.

In summary, the science of "original" medicine finds its roots and power in the Creator and Sustainer of all life on our small planet. God can do everything. When we put our trust and energy into learning the concepts and principles of His laws of health, He will bless us with healing knowledge, wisdom, and power. It is beyond our frail capabilities to learn these principles from any other source of knowledge outside of His approved methods.

I wish you health, happiness, and God's richest blessings as you pursue your goals to health and happiness for yourself, your family, your friends, your associates, and all those who come under your care and influence. To quote from our Source Book, the Bible, "Beloved, I pray that in all respects you may prosper and be in good health, just as your soul prospers." 3 John 2 NASB

BIBLIOGRAPHY

The Holy Bible	
Counsels on Diets and Foods	Ellen G. White
Counsels on Health	Ellen G. White
Healthful Living	Ellen G. White
Ministry of Health and Healing	Ellen G. White
Mind, Character, and Personality	Ellen G. White
The Medical Missionary Manual	Ellen G. White
Christian Temperance & Bible Hygiene	James and Ellen White
Drugs, Herbs and Natural Remedies	Mervin G. Hardinge, MD
CELEBRATIONS	General Conference of Seventh-day Adventists
Proof Positive	Neil Nedley, MD
Basic Principles of Total Health	Jim Sharps, N.D., H.D., Dr. NSc., Ph.D.
Medical Language	Susan Turley
Diet and Health Scientific Perspectives	Walter J. Veith
The Genesis Conflict	Walter J. Veith
The Genes of Genesis	Walter J. Veith
The Divine Prescription and Science of Health and Healing	Gunther Paulien, PhD
Google and Internet	

www.ingramcontent.com/pod-product-compliance
Lightning Source LLC
Chambersburg PA
CBHW041427270326
41932CB00030B/3488